Reality GP

Dr Ken B. Moody

Reality GP

Matador
5 Weir Road
Leicester LE8 0LQ
Tel: (+44) 116 2792299
Email: books@troubador.co.uk
Web: www.troubador.co.uk/matador

www.RealityGP.co.uk

9781848762190

Cover photo: www.Trahenna.com and Biggar Museums Trust.

Typeset in 11pt Stempel Garamond by Troubador Publishing Ltd, Leicester, UK
Printed in the UK by TJ International, Padstow, Cornwall

Matador is an imprint of Troubador Publishing Ltd

To friends, family and other patients.

Reviews of *View from the Surgery*

"Floating in the vitreous of his seen-it-all eyes and etched in skin exposed to years of hard work and dedication, he has captured general practice in all its complexity and uncertainty."
Dr Jill Murie, *Scottish Medical Journal*

"Like James Herriot with humans."
Fred MacAulay, BBC Radio Scotland

"It is hoped that these anecdotes are just the tonic for readers."
The Scots Magazine

"Disenchanted with our health care? Despairing there's no common sense left in the world? Take two stories, three times a day until negative feelings disappear."
Shari Low, *Daily Record*

"Lovely insights and all very recognizable."
Carl Whitehouse, retired Professor of General Practice, Manchester University

"It made me smile."
Lorraine Kelly, GMTV

Encompassing all the frustrating, funny, bizarre and down right stupid things that we have to contend with as doctors. But also touches on the difficulties common to all humanity and gives an insight to how we might face these. A great read."
Dr Des Spence, *British Medical Journal*

"As sharp as a scalpel and as comforting as Calpol: an excellent read."
Karen Hussain

"If only more GPs were like Dr Moody. This one is better than a sick line, an improvement on a prescription and the kind of paperback which might do you an injury if you read it in bed. You could hurt yourself laughing so much that you'd be in danger of falling out."
Alex Dickson. Smooth FM

CONTENTS

FOREWORD

Neither Dr Moody or I could have predicted that, little over a year after the publication of *View from the Surgery*, there would have been the demand (let alone the appetite) amongst readers for a second volume of his tales and anecdotes. I never had any doubt there would be sufficient material and, as we've both always maintained, the surgery is an endless source of material worth preserving for posterity and amusement, even within the bounds of confidentiality.

How one judges success never particularly troubled us, but we were uncertain whether there would be a readership sufficiently motivated to return to a book, that was never designed to be read at the one sitting. People seem to prefer endless sagas about others' lives and problems, whether real or otherwise. Authors, even before Dickens, were fully aware of this and wrote accordingly, often in installments, keeping readers on the edges of their seats.

In these increasingly busy and hectic times, most bibliophiles say they wish to be captivated by, or escape to, a world conjured up by the imagination of an author. Dr Moody claims very little in the way of imagination, originality or creativity and prefers to consider his writings as recordings of actual consultations and events, albeit from his rather wry perspective. As he once remarked: "My patients are rarely dull folk and certainly more colourful than their old, grey physician-and I don't mean in a jaundiced, cyanotic, plethoric or pallid sort of way!"

Publishers were generally impressed by the sales of "View" but remained a little unconvinced that a book written by a doctor that does not remotely resemble an academic tome, family medical book or murder mystery with a dysfunctional central character, appeals to a wider audience.

I do not purport to describe this book as even a modest contribution to the literature and it counts among those rejected by the posher publishing houses. The usual reason given was that a series of articles previously appearing in newspapers, over many years, does not necessarily come together naturally as a book. One languid, cheroot-smoking (though he was quickly asked to extinguish it!) fellow of some literary influence told me in a restaurant on George Street, that both books "are rather too much for one's senses to take in." I agreed, to the extent that they are indeed an eclectic mix of subjects and patients, but argued that this is a fair representation of an average day in general practice, as I know it. Doctors have to learn to adapt to dealing with life and death matters one minute, followed by indignant patients kept waiting with their crinkly toenails, the next. Perhaps I am the Watson to his Holmes and I have heard Dr Moody rue the fact that nowadays patients are often not apportioned the time they deserve. We would love to have the luxury of time to deliberate, like the great detective himself when he declared: "It is quite a three-pipe problem, and I beg that you won't speak to me for fifty minutes."

Each of these thousand-word essays, or chapters, takes almost exactly as long to read as a standard consultation lasts. Dr Moody could not readily be regarded as modern and rarely watches TV, but in some ways he writes like a "Reality GP." I believe he invites us to sit in his chair, don his wire spectacles and enter into the fascinating world of general practice.

It has been obvious to me that the quality of Ken's writing has improved. The old fellow was always a bit more than semi-literate but he seems to have gained a poetry to his pen, a vocation for his vocabulary and a niche for his narration. (Such clichéd alliteration is perhaps illustrative of why I am not a writer!) It is my considered opinion, however, that this book is at least as good as its predecessor but I am happy to let you, the reader, decide for yourself.

Whether this book should be seen as a sequel, a prequel or the potential script for a long-running radio drama, I do not know, but there seemed rather less for me to do in the preparation and, consequently, I declined to take credit for its editing. If there is ever a third volume, I suspect I will be asked politely to take a seat in the waiting room.

The marketing of the first book was an unanticipated pleasure. Doctors are not natural salespeople. I think we are generally too modest and reserved to promote products; and Scottish medics probably to an even greater degree. Doctors in this country are not, of course, allowed to advertise their own services but find there is rarely the need. Patients are rarely slow to seek us out in surgery.

Much was learned in the months following the release of *View from the Surgery* but, more importantly, tremendous fun was had all round. The chapter Selling One's Book within these pages gives a certain insight into this.

Once again, I urge readers not to attempt to "experience" all these chapters at the one sitting. Doctors tend to restrict ourselves to a dozen or so patients per surgery but sometimes obligingly allow a few more to be added. If it all gets a little too much, stop, breathe deeply and go and make yourself a cup of tea. There will always be cases waiting for you when you get back and there is often benefit in seeing things afresh. No matter how familiar you think you are with the human condition, like your attentive and kindly GP, you will never fail to be surprised.

David Carvel
Biggar 2009

PART 1

BEHIND THE SURGERY DOOR

BEING DETACHED

"How do you detach yourself from being affected by the tragedies and upsets your patients suffer, Dr Ken?" It was a question I get asked and wonder myself sometimes as to the answer. Ms Hart, as a patient and as a person, always took things personally and would be deeply affected by the misfortunes that life threw. You could almost say that Olive-May Hart wore her heart on her sleeve. She had been in nursing for a year or two but found the "emotional" side of things too troubling. She herself had indeed endured an astonishing catalogue of personal and family illness and loss but was finally reaching the end of her tether.

It is true that doctors are renowned for their apparent ability to remain calm and focused, even under the most trying of circumstances. Blood, guts and gore generally don't turn doctors' stomachs. We may be witness to the appalling consequences of: sustained, isolated or random assault; domestic violence; marital breakdown; childhood cancers; road accidents; parental neglect or indifference; elder abuse; the violation of housebreaking; rape; unfair dismissal; vexatious complaint; malicious gossip; grievous bodily harm; financial debt and repossession; drug and alcohol addiction; sudden or unexplained death and murder and suicide. The average general practitioner may not, of course, have to deal with the aftermath of all of these in a single week or even in a year but could almost certainly recall involvement with patients subject to each or several of these.

There is no doubt, we see the best and worst in people and human nature in this job. I am sure the police, fire and ambulance services could say the same but medics are in a fairly unique position where we see and help people through the initial, middle and later stages of crisis and suffering. We know how difficult anniversaries, Christmases and "would have been" birthdays are, when loss has been experienced. Sometimes we are best to just sit back and listen but we have to be vigilant for developing depression or other illnesses.

Doctors are not social workers, counsellors or an advice bureau. We cannot find accommodation, befriend, provide transport, ensure maximum benefits and entitlements or be a voice on the end of the phone in the middle of the night. Those who have tried have not been able to sustain such benevolence, have ultimately caused disappointment or had advantage taken of their good natures. But most importantly, it has meant other patients have not been given due time and attention. I cannot allow my mind to wander when the very next patient may be brewing their own illness or crisis. I cannot pretend though that some cases don't affect me deeply. I may lie in bed staring at the cobwebs in the cornice or find myself mulling over whether I might not have acted differently in surgery. Perhaps I should have read between the lines where physical illness was a manifestation of deeper emotional pain or I might have offered a more empathetic or kindly word of advice.

I think the crucial element to surviving as a doctor is to have a degree of emotional detachment. It would be entirely unfair to my family were I to return home each evening wrecked from what I had seen and heard that day in surgery. I cannot weep buckets for patients. It would be unfair on other patients if my bin was full of my moist paper hankies by ten o'clock each morning. I must remain objective and impartial. This can be difficult if I have known a family for years or their children are similar ages to my own. It may seem a little selfish, but this misfortune is not involving "my own." Perhaps

I would go to pieces if personal tragedy struck, I do not know, but until then I shall try to remain detached.

Being emotionally detached does not imply a lack of care or compassion but rather a true professionalism.

Sorry, Olive-May Hart, it might not answer your question but how can I help you today?

ROLLING OUT THE RED CARPET

"Well, if I have to wait six months for an appointment to see a specialist I'll just go privately," declared Mrs V. Eigh-Peegh resolutely. She asked if her wish met with any ethical objection on my part. Referring outwith the NHS goes against the weave for some of my colleagues, but I see no conflict of interest. I reassured Violet that she need not fear a verbal carpeting from me but nor should she expect a crimson woven pile to be rolled out on her behalf. It is not everyone in the practice who has the means to make such a decision to go privately. If a patient chooses to self fund, in some ways she is lightening the burden on the NHS. I do decline when asked , however, to refer simultaneously within both systems.

In a sense though, medicine used to be an entirely private affair. Years ago, all doctors were paid directly by their patients, rather than by the state through taxation. In poorer areas doctors' invoices, even for basic services, might not be affordable to many. Most kindly physicians wrote these off or even added a little to their wealthier clients' bills. But not all doctors took such a charitable or means-tested approach and some communities would have received little or no decent medical care. The introduction of the NHS sought to rid the nation of such treatment inequalities and the aim was that everyone would receive care depending solely on their needs, rather than on what they could afford.

After this enormous and commendable development, private medicine was perceived as being superfluous, but a luxury and privilege of the wealthy. Swanky hospitals were quiet, serene places and one was given as much (or more!) time and attention as was felt deserved.

Those who conceived and founded the NHS could never have imagined the health needs and demands of a litigious, consumer society little over half a century later. High tech scans and procedures and an ever aging and dependent population have put pressures on the system that could not have been foreseen. In some ways, it is also a victim of its own success. It is my belief that the increasing budgetary requirements to fund the NHS are unsustainable. I suspect a general insurance scheme, similar to that operating in other countries, will be adopted. Such systems are not flawless, as some people cannot obtain insurance at affordable premiums and may be little better "covered" than their predecessors. This is one of the reasons I remain a strong supporter of the NHS, but know that fundamental policy changes need to occur. These are too important to be left to the politicians though.

What many private patients forget is that the consultants they attend are the same doctors who work in NHS hospitals. The law tightly restricts the proportion of time a doctor may work in the private sector. Some people seem to entertain the notion that a superior breed of clinician inhabits these medical mansions and sits idly (while cleaners shampoo the red carpet!) waiting to minister upon their special patients.

Nowadays, any minor celebrity thinks he has made the big time if invited to stride down the vermillion rug, cheered by a few fans and admirers. (The same ones who will likely metaphorically pull it from under his feet when the appeal fades!)

Violet received her expedited treatment but later discovered it was no better than her neighbour's. I am happy to refer patients privately, if that is what they request, but ensure they are under no illusions and do not see the floor covering, or any other part of the fabric, through rose-tinted spectacles.

A GOOD DAD

"The things she said about me during the divorce were hurtful. Apparently I am lazy, vindictive and mean. It was strong stuff for her to say she never loved me and that the relationship was a sham. Things have got even nastier, Dr Ken, with the custody battle and all. But the comment that wounded me most, and I think the judge believed her, was when she accused me of being a bad father." Pat Ternal's marriage had disintegrated long before the decree absolute was signed. He and May had remained under the same roof for a few years, for the sake of their two young sons, but they both knew it was never going to work. "Amicable" would not be a word ever used to describe their separation.

Both Pat and his ex had each moved on to new relationships, though Pat recently found himself single again. This was only further ammunition and declared as evidence that he was "unstable and incapable of forming lasting and loving relationships."

Pat accepted mothers usually win custody, in all but the most exceptional circumstances, but only wanted to see and spend time with Vic and Tim as often as he could. May Ternal not only wanted to limit Pat's access to the minimum but sought to cut him out of their lives entirely.

I had known them both for some years and indeed May once consulted me about "Pat's unreasonable behaviour." He had apparently threatened her with violence or even resorted to a push, she showed me the bruises. If this truly occurred it was unacceptable but she was keen to inform the appointed social worker and me that "this is what the monster is capable of." I suspect, as is often the case, we were simply getting two sides to the one story, neither of which was particularly accurate.

Pat's reason for visiting me today was to ask for a character reference. Before I decided whether to oblige we discussed who were the real victims and biggest losers-the children.

What or who is a good dad, we mused? A good father is surely one who does his best for his kids. He may not be there all the time, for reasons of work or other circumstances, but he provides and cares for his offspring. He is patient and will make sacrifices of his time. He may find himself forgoing golf or residential weekends to sit through swimming or ballet lessons (he may partake if he wishes!) He may not get to read the newspaper when princesses have to be rescued from towers or spacemen from their alien captors. He shares his children's enthusiasm for learning and discovery. He sets a good example by being a reasonable, decent and honest chap. He is consistent, perhaps predictable, but never boring. He does not over-indulge or show addictive behaviour. He does not flare up at the merest provocation or storm off huffily. I believe he does not curse or even mutter expletives, at least not in their presence. He helps his kids explore the world and their own environment with respect and enthusiasm. He gives them opportunities that he himself may have been denied. He keeps them free from danger but still able to play to an extent that may result in bumps and scrapes. He knows to say "no" when malign influence or just being spoilt threatens. He encourages their friendship with others and is sociable with other parents, even when they share few other common interests or bring up their children differently. Even if he and mum have lost their love for each other this is never obvious, he knows how perceptive kids are. They may live apart but access and hand-overs, whether formal or informal, go smoothly. Parents should not strive to "outtreat" or outdo each other nor seek fault in the other's handling of illness or crisis. Above all, the kids are not used as weapons. In an ideal world children would be brought up by mum and dad but this is not and cannot always be the case.

Pat is not without his faults, he would readily agree. They have hardly set a good example of ideal parenting so far and lasting damage may have been done. I do believe Pat loves his kids and does his best for them and I know they adore him. I wrote him a letter of support, declaring him a good character, as far as I knew. We can only wait to see what happens.

A HIGH FEVER

The phone call came in at five minutes before six in the evening. It can be a little irritating when people leave it until the end of the working day before deciding to call the doctor. In this case though, Mrs Verre had been keeping an eye on, both her daughter Fiona and the mercury, rising and falling all day long. The fifteen-year-old had remained as hot and lethargic but was now "poorly responsive."

I could leave my supper to go cold but not my patient to further heat up. Many visits can safely wait until the following morning, and conditions often improve in the interim, but not when such dramatic symptoms are so clearly described.

Within twenty minutes I was standing in the young teenager's bedroom, surrounded by boy bands and worried family members (well, just posters of the former!) A hot looking Fi Verre was now shivering and had awoken on my arrival. She nodded off between my questions, but probably not this time from tedium. "She just won't drink either, doctor," added mum, though an unopened bottle of orangeade at her bedside told me as much. She went on, "It was her gran who reminded me that Fi was in Kenya last month. I don't think she took the tablets after she came home; in fact I know she didn't, here they are here." Examining the unopened silver foil packets, we concluded she could only have taken them for the duration of the trip, at best, and not for the required four weeks afterwards. Our travel clinic nurse, I know, would have emphasized this to Fi and her mum, but this was no time for blame.

I had visited, concerned that she might have been suffering meningitis or influenza but, in the light of this new information, malaria became the more likely diagnosis. I was pleased to note that she was a rather bright pink colour and not yellow from jaundice. Neither was she delirious but I expressed my concerns and went downstairs to telephone the infectious diseases on-call doctor.

Malaria (from the old Italian *mala aria*: bad air) has a global annual incidence of over 500 million people. Some 2 million, often young malnourished children, die from this insect-borne infectious disease. It is thought to have existed for as long as humankind has trodden the earth and some scientists postulate that malaria has been responsible for a greater number of deaths than any other disease or condition. Despite this, there is still no vaccine, only insecticides and many simply die through the lack of access to treatment and medical care.

Little Plasmodium parasites are carried by the female anopheles mosquito. She and all her sisters, aunts and nieces inject, usually sleeping, humans and other mammals with the infection and there it attacks and multiplies within red blood cells.

Fi Verre had visited her relations abroad before and, each time, they ensured she took her anti-malarials. They also insisted she slept within a fine-mesh net and routinely sprayed insecticide liberally before venturing out. Despite this, her young pale skin seemed particularly alluring to the murderous little blood suckers. By the time I saw her, the numerous bites to her shoulders and shins had faded but the damage had been been done; the infection acquired. Fi's diagnosis was confirmed at the infirmary, by the examination of a blood sample under the microscope. She was treated appropriately, recovered without event and was home the following week.

We don't get too many tropical diseases in these, more temperate, parts. International travel is increasingly common and people can inadvertently bring home more than just souvenirs. It is feared that climate change may radically alter the distribution of diseases, such as malaria. In Scotland, we're just plagued by midges in the summer and head lice all year round. Irritating, certainly, but never deadly.

This was my first case of malaria in general practice and hopefully will be my last. Fi learned the hard way about failing to appreciate her medication but is already planning her next African trip.

SANDS OF TIME

The sands of time are sinking, the dawn of Heaven breaks;
The summer morn I've sighed for-the fair, sweet morn awakes:
Dark, dark hath been the midnight, but dayspring is at hand
And glory, glory dwelleth in Immanuel's land.

These, of course, are the opening words to A R Cousin's powerful and stirring Victorian hymn "The Sands of Time are Sinking." They are still chosen for funerals and I first heard them at my grandfather's service. It is not usually recommended that all nineteen verses are sung on these occasions, as the sands indeed would be slipping away, for everyone else in attendance.

Anne Cousin (1824-1906) was the daughter of a Leith doctor and climbed just that one step higher up the ladder of respectability, by marrying a minister. She became the lady of the manse, in Melrose.

The accompanying music is uplifting but unattributed. This is widely regarded as Anne's finest and most memorable of her 107 hymns but, in truth, I always found the title rather fatalistic and doom-laden. I don't suppose nineteenth-century Presbyterianism was ever famed for its warm, comforting cosiness or ready reminders that life is for enjoying, rather than just enduring. Nowadays, we often take life for granted, as if it were only for pleasure. We cannot argue though that we are anything other than mortal. Each of us, like the very grains themselves, will one day pass away to that other level. (Some up-defying gravity-and some down, perhaps!)

But just supposing we were able to steal a glance at the hourglass and were given a fair idea when the said sands were due to "sink." Would we live life any differently? Would our priorities change? Would we do more for ourselves or for others, and for what would we wish to be best remembered ?

I knew a man who caught sight of the hourglass. Alexander Shore, in his middle years, was given a terminal diagnosis. He had only ever lived for himself and for the present time. His sole aim had been to make money; as much as possible, regardless of the means. This cost Sandy. It cost him many friends, his marriage (to June) and his integrity. He had not built his castle or his character on solid ground. On receipt of the news, he looked around and found he was all alone, marooned as it were; the proverbial island. In an instant, he was forced to reassess all that was important. Unlike the pharaohs in their sandy sarcophagi, he could not take his wealth with him and would look pretty ridiculous if he tried. Like the tide going out on him, he was left staring at the flotsam and jetsam of his life, washed up at his feet.

He saw the gritty reality of life for the first time. Sandy realized that all that was dear, he had let slip through his hands.

For the first time, his life started to take shape. June even came back. Like many people, he had lived only for the moment, failing to secure solid foundations of trust and love. How we wish to be remembered by friends and society at large is determined by the examples we set and impressions we make right now.

The sand itself serves as a reminder of the transience of life. This particulate matter may have started as rock but millennia of erosion and weathering leads to the eventual production of these, the smallest parts, as beautiful and unique as they are.

Ashes to ashes, dust to dust and sand to sand.

PAINTING IT BLACK

"You said mum only had a matter of weeks left but she lived a full four months. Why do you doctors always paint so black a picture?" asked Mrs Carr-Bonne.

One of the areas of general practice in which I feel least comfortable is when asked to quantify how long a patient has before she shuffles off the mortal coil. Ultimately, of course, it can only be the Giver and taker(s) of life who issue such specifics but doctors, having a better vantage point than most, could at least hazard an educated guess when pressed. I am not versed in the black arts, however, so cannot accurately predict the date of one's expiry. Were I to boldly state "six days, eight hours and thirteen minutes," it is likely that I would not be taken seriously or could reasonably be suspected of having a hand in the matter.

During the course of our medical education (which arguably ends only on retirement!) we learn about conditions, their treatments and the likely outcomes. Cardiovascular disease, cancers and the unrelenting "Anno Domini" are appreciated and respected for all that they are. Medical intervention can lessen the effects of disease and even defer death but we observe the general course of human illnesses from the privileged positions we occupy. Nobody's condition follows the textbooks to the letter, thank goodness, and the art of medicine is seeing and treating each patient on their own merits and in the individual context.

I'm not sure that we do paint predictably black pictures. We just sometimes impart bad news in an honest fashion, which may not be what people wish to hear. It would be unfair to roller the walls of wishful-thinking with white emulsion, by promising certain cure, when a somewhat darker prognosis is the reality. Our credibility is also at stake.

Sadly, we also find ourselves practising medicine in an increasingly defensive way. We are less likely to be sued for portraying a grimmer picture than events ultimately determined, than for giving a falsely bright one. Newspapers love to describe survivors as having "baffled the doctors" by outliving expectations. "Doctors only gave me 26 weeks but here I am 26 years later and training for my 26th marathon!"

But it is not just discussions about death that attract accusations of decorating in dark colours or painting with palettes of pitch. The course of unpredictable conditions like Multiple Sclerosis can be ones where it is difficult to offer advice. Nurses and doctors may feel less than helpful when repeatedly stating: "who knows what will happen next." General anaesthesics and concurrent illnesses are stresses on the body which may lead to relapses in MS. It seems reasonable to warn of such eventualities but this should not be interpreted as being negative, gloomy or black. Similarly, when a handicapped child is born into a family, as much support as possible should be offered. This should be in the form of encouragement and understanding but also by mentioning, when appropriate, possible limitations and expectations as life proceeds.

I believe there are varying shades of grey in the pictures we paint and outlooks we offer patients. It is rare for me not to give people any hope. I may not have seen a particular cure or even an improvement in all my years of practice, but that does not mean it cannot occur. I continue to be surprised at how patients defy all expectations. Even the deepest, darkest tunnels sometimes have light at the other end.

THE SNIP

It was only after some persuasion that the editor nodded his assent when I suggested I write about this rather "delicate subject." He seemed a little concerned that I might do so in too "anatomical" a fashion or litter the article with puns and innuendo. Really! As if I would! I argued that people nowadays are less sensitive souls than one might imagine and it can surely never be wrong to increase readers' knowledge and to banish a few misconceptions. He picked me up on this latter term, describing it as "Freudian," as by performing vasectomies it is conceptions that one is indeed trying to "miss." I do enjoy his sense of humour.

Cy Sawyers, an infrequent visitor to the surgery, told me he was attending having been sent along by his dear wife. They were in their early forties and considered their family, of two beautiful girls, to be complete. Neither of Siss's pregnancies had been straightforward and had both ended in Cesarean section. Cy could not argue that Siss had not done her bit for the family, and now it was his turn. I admire chaps who step up to the breech and drop their breeches, as it were (is that OK, Ed?) Many do not, even when they know that further pregnancies may be to the endangerment of their partner's life.

I always enquire whether a chap has had any relevant surgery previously, such as a hernia repair. I ensure he is aware of the nature of the actual procedure and that he knows he will be awake throughout, unless he is a quivering wreck. The surgeon then carefully shaves (after all they were originally barbers!) and injects local anaesthetic. He (or she!) then makes a small incision on either side and teases out the actual vas deferens. This is similar in diameter and colour to a piece of string. Previously, he would have deliberately burnt the left and right vas but now small sections are cut and sent to the laboratory (to ensure the correct bits have been removed!) He then folds back and ties the remaining severed ends to ensure never the twain shall meet. After that, the incisions are made good and the chap packed off for a cup of tea to whet his parched palate.

It is only fair to warn the responsible fellow that he will likely feel, for a few days afterwards, that he has ridden on horseback down the Grand Canyon. The bruising and tenderness may be quite impressive. Probably the most important piece of advice that can be given is that sterility does not occur at the time of the snip. Because the vas is such a tightly coiled structure, "little swimmers" can remain within and may do what nature intended, for up to several weeks. For this reason, a full two months must elapse, after which two specimens are submitted for analysis. With a nod that the "tadpoles" are truly absent, unprotected relations can occur. No technique is perfect and, as with any procedure, failure may result. By and large though, if there is a subsequent pregnancy, it is quite "conceivable" that there has been, shall we say, third party involvement.

It is also worthwhile informing couples that vasectomy is designed to be permanent. Circumstances can, of course, change but reversal is difficult and is not done on the NHS.

(It was once mischievously suggested the private surgeons only do these ops to "help make ends meet.") Generally, the longer it has been since the original procedure, the less likely attempted reversal is to be successful.

It is also for this reason, that I caution younger chaps against having the procedure. I recall one lad in his early twenties, already the father of two. I suggested that, as tired as he and his wife were with toddlers, their thoughts for additions may change at a later date.

True to form, nine months later, a baby boy entered the world and was amusingly named after their cautious "family doctor." I almost expected a request for maintenance for my paternalistic (but certainly not paternal!) role in the matter. I was happy to refer the contented young father for the snip soon after.

It was interesting to read that the first human vasectomy was performed in 1897. It is perhaps more curious, if not toe-curling, to learn that "experiments" had been occurring for over a century, leading up to this.

It is usually urologists who perform these relatively straightforward procedures, several times every week, but some GPs are keen to maintain their surgical skills and do one or two each lunchtime. I knew of one former colleague who claimed to have performed his own vasectomy, so he could "not blame any other blighter if it went wrong." Perhaps taking matters into his own hands a little too much.

There, I believe the editor cannot complain. I have written about vasectomy in as sterile a sort of way as I could.

COMFORTABLE DOCTOR

"And you just sit there on your fat....padded chair. You don't know what hard work, toil and struggle are really like. You doctors are all just the same!"

I'll spare you the details leading up to Mr Watt Stryfe's tirade but, other than to say, I still think he swings the lead and would not recognize heavy labour, or the said heavy metal, were it to hit him squarely between the eyes. I've provided him with medical certificates before but declared that, on this occasion, a twitchy eyelid fell below the threshold for genuine incapacity.

I felt neither sympathy or guilt as he slammed the door behind him. What I did ponder upon, though, was his assertion that my lot is a comfortable one compared with others in the workforce. Might he have a point, however indelicately expressed?

I would strongly disagree with his generalization that there is no variation in attitude or aptitude within the medical profession. I accept that being a maturing country physician, well established in the community, is not the world's most challenging occupation. You'll note, I do not speak for my beleaguered colleagues working in inner cities, prisons or war-torn areas, who are subject to quite different conditions and demands.

I don't mean to diminish my own responsibilities or appear flippant in this respect. My partners, here in the practice, may feel quite differently about their workloads (and my contribution!) and wish to beat a path to my door and a crater in my skull. I know I could make an error of judgement tomorrow that might be unforgivable and live with me for the rest of my days.

But, considering the rather predictable pattern to my day, I know I will see some three-dozen patients before nightfall. I can often anticipate the reasons for their visits and may actually have requested their attendance. If I am not on duty, I can walk to work; occasionally returning home for lunch and certainly for dinner. I can kick on my slippers and listen to the evening concert on the wireless, without interruption. I am under no obligation to work overnight or at weekends, so plan my leisure activities accordingly. I am not under constant threat of assault or injury at work and most members of the public treat me with reasonable respect (which I may not always be due!) I am not called to hurriedly-arranged meetings in places or countries in which I have no wish to go. I am not required to reapply for my position annually or prove my superiority over workmates before "efficiency cuts." My remuneration and superannuation arrangements are better than fair and my home will only be repossessed for reasons of my own fecklessness.

I am not thwarted and frustrated by a lack of medical supplies, resources or clean water. Food is plentiful and people tend to be over rather than under nourished. Deadly infectious diseases are rare and people are able to take responsibility for their own health. I have seen almost every medical condition and outcome at least once and know how people react to illness, loss and uncertainty. I know when to reassure, when to worry, when to seek advice and when to tell people to stop wasting their time and mine. I have seen wonder drugs and treatments come and go. I have made myself unpopular by insisting on patients' readmission to hospital after premature discharge. I have been both overcautious and under attentive in my assessments and diagnoses. I have spoken when I shouldn't and been silent when intervention was necessary. I write my opinions (for that is all they are!) without persecution and am subject only to gentle criticism!

Throughout my medical career, I have tried to learn from my own and others' mistakes and inexperience and hope to manage new issues and challenges appropriately.

I don't think I take my relative comfort for granted, do I?

STARTIN' STATINS

I have no immediate plans to make tape/disc recordings for the benefit of my patients (certainly not of me singing!) If I were so inclined, it would have to be of my lipid lecture (my statin speech): the conversations I have about cholesterol blood test results. More than any other topic, I find myself either in surgery or on the telephone, discussing these numbers and what, if anything, ought to be done to address the situation.

I have been in medical practice long enough to remember how irrelevant we once considered our circulating blood fat levels to be. Indeed, eating lard was considered healthy and fashionable. I recall an advertisement featuring a bright young family, stepping through the waves, under the caption: "They're happy because they eat lard!" There was nothing subtle of subliminal; eat fat and you will feel and look good! If you happened to suffer a heart attack or a stroke, you were just dashed unlucky. Despite such dubious advice, people in the post war period lived generally healthier lives than we do now. They exercised more and ate less. Old black and white footage of beach scenes show crowds of slim people. Revisit these same shores (if there is not a pollution warning!) and you will be left in little doubt that our population is becoming fatter. The concern about cholesterol is that it forms fatty streaks within the blood vessel walls. (Such "fatty streaks" should not be confused with overweight people propelling themselves indecently down the beach!)

The relationship between blood pressure, smoking and cholesterol levels, with one's health and mortality, is now considerably clearer. People are better informed about these risk factors and it seems, almost everyone has knowledge or an opinion about their cholesterol.

Were I to actually dial a patient at home and, as soon as he answered, press "play," I suspect my credibility would sink even further than that of a telesales cold-caller offering to sell double glazing as one sits down to dinner. My conscience would not allow me to practise the art of medicine in this way. I presume, our professional judge, jury and executioner, the General Medical Council, would forbid such methods anyway but, as medicine becomes increasingly impersonal, I rather expect to hear such advice coming from the government soon. If "listeners" had any questions, they might be directed to the internet: a ready source of information, but often itself of questionable quality!

Many people believe, erroneously, that their lipid profile is a barometer of their eating habits. Very few claim, or admit, to eat poorly but acknowledge they sometimes "lapse" or are partial to the odd treat. By and large, one's genetics have a greater bearing on the numbers and levels than the quality of one's diet, but that is not to say nothing can be done.

Research suggests, it is in one's best interests to have a "Total cholesterol" of under five (mmol/L) It is this particular reading that enquirers tune in to but this is only one element of the equation. So called "good" and "bad" cholesterols (HDL and LDL respectively) and the Triglyceride level all have a bearing in one's overall cardiovascular "risk." There then comes the decision whether or not to reach for the prescription pad. Other medicines have come and gone in the treatment of hyperlipidaemia but, by far, the Statin group is the most effective. These drugs are widely appreciated and patients often have their own firm views on their use. As a pharmaceutical agent they are certainly not without possible problems and side-effects. I often say (but not currently on any tape!) that if they and anti-inflammatory medicines had fewer associated problems my life, as a prescriber, would be considerably easier. Statins, in as many as 15% of all people, cause unacceptable aches and pains. This may not be immediately apparent and I've sometimes advised folk, after taking them for years, that their "arthritis" may in fact be statin-induced. When successfully established on a statin, once or twice-yearly blood tests are recommended and tweaking the dose or changing from one statin to another may be necessary.

It is remarkable quite how significantly busier the surgery has become in recent years. Much of this is due to the monitoring and discussion of cholesterol and its treatment.

Perhaps in the waiting room I should broadcast, in an Orson Welles fashion, a fearsome warning. Not that the Martians have landed but, for those with uncontrolled cholesterols, there is an equally imminent threat of "interplanetary transfer." Better not, I'll stick with the given facts and deal with each person on their own merits.

THE WISHING CHAIR

I never met Mrs Gyffte, the grandmother of a good friend. She spent the last few years of her life in a nursing home. Her son and the rest of the family knew it was the level of care she required but always felt the actual care was less than might reasonably have been expected. When she died, in her ninetieth year, they were a little taken aback to be given forty-eight hours to clear her room of its effects.

The distinct impression was that the proverbial eye was on the clock and the next income-generating client was waiting to be wheeled in. Had things been handled rather more sensitively, I suspect the Gyfftes would have been happy for her furniture to remain for the use of other residents (and this would have been physically easier) but that was not to be.

Mrs Gyffte had benefited from the use of a comfortable reclining chair. It was on this expensive, cushioned and electrically operated item that their late and beloved relative had spent much of her last few months, and the family now wished to pass it on. It remained in immaculate condition.

The family approached me in my capacity as a (but not her) general practitioner, asking if I knew of an elderly or disabled person in the community who might benefit from the recliner. Nobody sprang to mind. (I suppose if one was capable of "springing" then such a chair might not be necessary!) I consulted our district nursing colleagues, knowing they not only visit more homes than I but also patients in neighbouring practices. One wit amongst them asked if the colour might blend well with her own fireside furniture. I suggested it might but the Gyfftes would not look too favourably on such snaffling and misappropriation.

By the good fortune that can sometimes be taken as providence, the very next day I was called to visit an elderly gentleman. I had not needed to visit or even think of Mr Elder for sometime but did so as I drove out to his rather distant village. His frailty and slowness were becoming rather extreme and his mobility, consequently, was greatly impaired. On this occasion it was a chest infection that demanded my medical attention but I noticed the double-cushioned, wooden-armed, upright chair upon which he perched. Yes, it was a worry to him he said, particularly when manoeuvring stiffly from his zimmer frame to this lightweight chair. It often rocked back to a perilous angle, apparently, when he landed heavily on it.

I mentioned the existence and offer of the recliner chair and how I felt it might be a suitable replacement for the aging one he currently used. Mr Elder seemed rather uncertain as to why his doctor should have become a furniture salesman. I was quick to reassure him that the Gyffte family was wishing to gift the chair to a person who had similar needs to their late (grand)mother. He appreciated this but expressed the concern that he would be unable to match such generosity and charity in his lifetime. I reassured him that the family only sought someone else's comfort and safety, nothing else. He smiled his assent and I think my eyes may have been as moist as his.

The following evening, Mrs Gyffte's son and I drove the recliner to its new home. (As sophisticated as the chair is, it is only electrically operated and not petrol driven and so we had to strap it to a car roof rack!) Mr Elder's daughter was there on our arrival and guided us as we carried the heavy item from car, through the narrow mid-terrace doorway, to its new resting place. Mr Elder watched from the relatively safe distance of the kitchenette as we defied the laws of Geometry; negotiating lintels, standard lamps and paintwork. Both families expressed their gratitude to each other and to me but I wouldn't entertain the latter. I was only a facilitator for the good deeds of others. The polite offer of money was made but the genuine need and evident pleasure were more than sufficient. If the Elder family really wished to make a gesture, we learned that Mrs Gyffte's preferred charity in her later life was Rachel House, the children's hospice. If desired, a modest donation could be sent to that most worthy cause in Kinross.

The chair, as practical and comfortable as it is, carries the good wishes from one older person's family to another by way of seriously ill children.

HANGING UP THE KEYS

There are few subjects in general practice (and perhaps in life!) that inspire such passionate debate as that of drivers and when to hang up the keys for the last time. As the price of fuel continues to rise and our roads become ever more congested, alternative means of transport become more attractive but I really refer to that increasingly populous, vocal and empowered group; the elderly, and elderly drivers in particular.

I am often consulted by relatives, concerned that dad stubbornly remains behind the wheel when it is evident he ought not to be. He may indeed have flown in the Battle of Britain but that does not necessarily imply, six or seven decades later, he retains such skill and dexterity at ground level. Most of us can readily think of family members or neighbours who drove (or still drive) when common sense suggests this to be dodgy.

"Should his doctor not have spoken to him before now?" Well, often doctor has but the advice was not heeded, or was inaccurately relayed back to the family. In my experience, such patients rarely consult their GPs, without encouragement or even coercion.

I suspect most older drivers know when best to give up or can be gently persuaded but I remain concerned about those who lack the ability to make this call. I remember one lady who consulted me on other matters but brought the subject around to her driving. It was my considered opinion that the time had indeed, regretfully, come when she should park the car for the last time. She thanked me for my "great sensitivity and judgement" and I felt some satisfaction at the outcome. I mentioned her sometime later to my colleagues only to discover she had consulted us all in recent months-and still hadn't got the answer she wanted to hear! There surely has to be a more robust system than this.

At present, the DVLA asks all new septuagenarians (and on every third birthday thereafter) to declare whether one suffers any medical conditions likely to impair the ability to drive. Superficially, that is commendable but it relies entirely on one's insight, honesty and objectivity. People may simply fail to recognize that their tremor, arthritis or forgetfulness compromise their ability to drive safely. There is a fine imposed on those who make fraudulent statements or withhold information but it is those with physical frailties, general slowing or early dementias who, even from a doctor's point of view, are more difficult to assess.

When I offer my views on issues of driving and the elderly, critics are quick to comment that it is young, inexperienced drivers who cause more serious accidents. Numerically, this is correct and I would report an idiot on wheels when I saw one.

There are very few medical conditions unique to older people but many that are commoner. Younger sufferers of, say, stroke should be and are judged by the same criteria as the elderly.

Only twice have I notified the DVLA of my serious concerns about patients and their driving. In the first case, a man in his 40s deliberately failed to inform the Agency that he had suffered his first epileptic fit in many years. I had ensured he was aware that the law clearly states one cannot drive until seizure-free for twelve months. When I saw him dropping off his children at school I was left with no option. The second case was an elderly lady who latterly was negotiating roundabouts in the wrong direction and demolishing fences on a regular basis. She could no more navigate her way home from the shops than she could walk to the post box. I suppose I wrote the letter for her, knowing she never would. I appreciate there are issues of confidentiality but I believe these are overridden by concerns for public and personal safety.

My contention is, rather than the simple licence reapplication that currently exists, drivers should undergo regular, medical assessments. I accept 70 is a somewhat arbitrary age but would seem to be a reasonable place to start. I suggest, though, it is not one's own GP who is given this responsibility. We are quite busy enough with clinical and administrative work but, more importantly, we are probably not objective enough. Living and working in this small rural community, I am not afraid to admit that I might be too soft. Access to a car, even for short trips, often keeps an older person functioning but may still present unacceptable dangers. Call me lily (or anything else!) livered but I might be swayed by bottles gifted every Christmas or by tearful pleas. On the other hand, a negative decision may mar a long-established professional relationship and a patient may fail to seek help in real time of need.

I am not calling for compulsory driving tests, with all the stresses that would bring (nor because I would likely fail were I to sit one tomorrow!) I am suggesting the introduction of a universal and fair assessment at an independent medical level. That's not too radical is it?

DOCTORS WHO KILL

Primum non nocere, translated for non-classicists like myself, is closest in meaning to: "First do no harm." Contrary to popular belief, this phrase is not part of the Hippocratic Oath but is often used as a guiding principle by practising doctors and medical ethicists. It reminds us that, when considering and selecting treatment for a patient, we ought to recognize and weigh up the potential risks against the anticipated benefits. The risks, for all but the simplest of treatments, can ultimately be grave.

There have been several doctors who clearly did not abide by this maxim and are consequently remembered for all the wrong reasons. Negligence and incompetence will usually lead to one's summons before the General Medical Council but will rarely lead to criminal charges. There are those few malign individuals, however, who may be skilled and competent in their practise of everyday medicine but deliberately take life for reasons beyond the comprehension of colleagues and society in general.

I confess to now spending much of my life in this small, square room, dwelling on my past actions and imaging how it must be in the outside world. To brighten my day, I get visitors who have to check-in first at the main desk. Fortunately, the parallels between incarceration and my inclination-to be a GP-end there!

Dr Harold Shipman is the best known and most recently convicted doctor. He is in fact the only British doctor to be found guilty of murdering his patients, though several others have been charged and acquitted, or found guilty of other serious crimes. It has even been suggested that Shipman may be the most prolific serial killer in history. Books have been written and will continue to be published about this nefarious medical practitioner and his dubious legacy. The ramifications of his appalling crimes will last for at least another generation.

Other doctors in years gone by almost captured the nation's attention to the same degree. John Bodkin Adams (1899-1983) was convicted on thirteen counts of prescription fraud and falsifying forms, including cremation certificates, but never of murder. One-hundred and sixty of his patients died under suspicious circumstances. There seemed to be an obvious motive when it emerged over 80% of these trusting souls had mentioned him in their wills.

Dr Crippen (1862-1910) is a name familiar to most. He was an American-born homeopathist convicted of the poisoning and burying of his wife's body in his London garden. Perhaps it was his dramatic attempt to flee to Canada with his mistress and his arrest being the first made with the aid of wireless communication that drew such attention and notoriety.

The murdering medic who probably intrigues me the most is Edward Pritchard (1825-1865) perhaps it is because he had Scottish connections. He poisoned his wife and mother-in-law with Antimony and almost certainly their servant girl too, though the evidence for the teenager's murder proved insufficient. He was the last person to be publicly hanged in Glasgow.

William Palmer (1824-1856) seemed to poison almost everyone to whom he owed money or those whose insurances were in his favour. Being one of his patients, ironically, was a safer bet then being of his acquaintance, though his medical abilities were said to have been questionable.

I could find no record of a female doctor being charged or convicted of murder but shall, of course, continue my reading. What I did conclude is that these contemptible figures were simply murderers who happened to be doctors. They should not be allowed to bring the medical profession into disrepute or to pave the way to over-regulation and stifling monitoring of the medical profession. These killers attained positions with the highest level of trust in society and then proceeded to grossly abuse the privilege using their acquired skills and knowledge. Poisoning was almost always the method of dispatch and financial benefit the commonest motive. Psychopathic tendencies could be seen in some of them, but not all.

Fortunately, on the whole, this gruesome contingent did not escape justice; but these are only the ones we know about. There may be others who evaded detection. Cremation is literally a burning of the evidence but with burial the evidence lies dormant. John Bodkin Adams largely escaped justice and even managed to have himself reinstated on the medical register. This was despite his fraudulence and the strong suspicion he had killed scores of people. Even after his trial, curiously, some of his patients continued to consult him, such was the trust and faith he had engendered.

There have been other doctors, such as David Moor (1947-) who admitted to helping many of his patients die. Each of these patients had a terminal condition and he maintained he was only ending, with consent, their suffering. Ironically, it was during Adams' trial that the principle of Double Effect was established. This is where a doctor, genuinely attempting to relieve pain in a sufferer, may unintentionally shorten life. Euthanasia continues to be a hotly debated subject but must be clearly distinguished from cold-blooded murder.

After such convictions, lessons are learned, necessary changes made and controls tightened-but these must never be for political expediency, only for the safety of the public. Shipman is probably not the last in the line of murderous doctors but it is unlikely crimes of that scale will be seen again.

PART 2

MEDICAL MUSINGS

THE COLUMN

Well, well. Two whole years have passed since I embarked on the adventure of becoming a columnist. One-hundred and four articles have appeared in print and if you have bothered to read more than one or two of them, I congratulate and thank you.

The editor of this august newspaper requested, through the diligent services of Ms Freya Lanss, that I pen a few notes each week about my experiences, thoughts and views and so *View from the Surgery* was born. I feared I would not find much worthwhile to record and what I might consider meaningful may be bound by rules of confidentiality. Initially begrudgingly and latterly willingly, I set about the task. I never wanted to write in a dry and purely informative way. Others have done, and still do, this far better than I ever could. I also read too many dull columns in "nationals" each weekend to write in such a fashion. I believe laughter is the best medicine and the best medicine is laughter, except perhaps for antibiotics.

I use the precious column inches afforded to me each week to express myself and write in what is intended to be an amusing way. Some have not shared in this humour and objected, most notably to my lack of political correctness. I confess to finding my musings therapeutic and refreshing and perhaps even cathartic. As I sit in surgery listening to Earnest Dawdler and others spout forth in a style that will never raise my enthusiasm or even when Cyrus Lyell's condition demands all my attention and ministrations, I often wonder whether readers would wish to "spectate." The overwhelming opinion seems to be, yes. All patients mentioned (or those who would recognize themselves!) have given their expressed consent or tacit approval. The others would probably nod from beyond the grave.

I do not list "Columnist" next to "General Practitioner" on my business card. In truth, my card is so dog-eared and I attend too few grand functions to require one these days. I am also well kent enough to those who need to know who I am.

After a few months of column writing, I felt a little photograph or image might add to each piece. The first was of the great author John Buchan, taken in fact from an old cigarette card. These pictures, I admit, can be of varying interest. One was of rhubarb stalks and leaves and I content myself that I am unlikely to run out of material if I can dedicate a whole article to this tasty plant. I have no current plans for one about custard however.

The column could never have continued without the helpful suggestions and contributions of readers. Several ideas have been adopted and, after consultation, adapted. The photographs sent to me have varied from the gorgeous to the grotesque. (To one contributor's disappointment, the feature on hemorrhoids will have to wait.) I was obliged to return another photo to a certain lady declaring that, as she should well know, I remain happily married. Yet another reader offered to nominate me for local newspaper columnist of the year. I was most touched that my views and ramblings might be considered anything other then irrelevant drivel but on discovering that no such award exists took this to be either spoof or misguided flattery.

I do not write this column for any commercial purpose and have turned down several offers of sponsorship. It is probably unseemly for physicians to have affiliations to the trades or other professions, but I gave each offer due consideration. I felt local plumbers might imply too Urological a bent to my writings and posh restaurants, though delightful places, are too upmarket for one who indulges in fish suppers occasionally, after difficult late evening surgeries.

Mrs Eva Rywurd claims never to have missed an article and is quick to point out apparent inconsistencies. I once made reference to a discussion with my erstwhile colleague, Dr Bodie Aiken, after doing a feature on his retirement. I can of course still seek counsel from this wise old gent but, Eva was right, I should have been more careful with the order in which articles are submitted.

So, two years down and who knows how long to go. There is no doubt the breadth and depth of subject matter each week in surgery could keep this column going ad infinitum (rather then ad nauseum I hope!) I cannot say, but with your ongoing support and comments we could have one or two more anniversaries yet.

SIGNIFICANT BIRTHDAYS

For some, birthdays are to be celebrated enthusiastically particularly when divisible by ten, for others they are not.

Mr Sykes Tighe fell firmly into the latter category. Being rather less firm, on a more delicate matter, he visited me one day in surgery. I questioned and examined him and felt that he seemed in fairly sound health. I explained that anxiety can interfere with one's performance in that department and asked if the nervous expression he wore was for good reason. His good lady once again, as with every significant birthday since his eighteenth, had insisted on throwing him a party. He was fast approaching the end of another decade and knew that again the glasses would be chinking, the helium balloons inflated and the novelty cake baked. These were becoming increasing large gatherings as the family and circle of friends widened. Ironically, Mr Tighe was a shy chap by nature and never enjoyed being the centre of such attention. He hated making speeches on demand, could hardly hear a thing above background chatter and champagne only gave him indigestion. He knew such admissions would sadden his wife, especially after all her considerable organizational efforts. He just never managed to express his preference for a simpler, humbler affair, such as a candlelit dinner for two. I suspect this was the silent wish he made when instructed, after blowing out his candles. If so, it never came true. Having attended his previous celebration, this post-puff pause seemed to get lengthier, but perhaps with advancing years he just takes longer to get his breath back.

Most cultures celebrate the anniversaries of one's birth. Some religious sects refuse to acknowledge them, believing there to be some pagan significance.

The Jewish faith celebrates the bar mitzvah when a boy turns thirteen and the bat mitzvah when his sister reaches twelve. In the West, the eighteenth and twenty-first birthdays are regarded as "coming of age" and rather arbitrarily declared dates when one acquires the wisdom and responsibility to be able to vote and raise a glass in celebration. By thirty, people have generally flown the nest and found a soulmate, perhaps having already become parents themselves. Dinners with other tired parents are the norm. Forty tends to see an acceptance of middle-age and the realization that sporting and other dreams might never be met. Fifty may be more modestly acknowledged as the children are increasingly expensive to maintain and are horrified that mum or dad would even consider declaring to the world that they are "so ancient." Sixty may be combined with a retiral do but, as the pension pot diminishes, this may not occur for another ten or twenty years! Ninety, and particularly one-hundred, are marvelous reasons for celebration, usually prompted by the now elderly surviving offspring, if mum feels fit and able to attend. Beyond that, of course, there are few birthdays but, as the population generally ages, Her Majesty may be subject to repetitive strain injury, signing all these telegrams.

Some wag once compared life to an orchestra. He declared that it matters not how long one plays, but how well. This has a discordant ring of truth about it when hearing an amateur musical production giving little enthusiasm to stay beyond the interval but, when experiencing the harmonious heavenly music of the National Orchestra, we willingly shout "Encore."

I suggested to Mr Sykes Tighe that he is in pretty good health but, by definition, cannot have too many more significant "decade" birthdays to endure. Curiously, he seemed to take consolation in this fact. He knows he continues to be in the fortunate position where he is loved and appreciated and can celebrate the passing of another ten years of good health. I prescribed him an antacid medication to keep things down but advised against anything that may have the opposite effect elsewhere.

On the next occasion we met, the smile was back and he told me the fizz was too. The corks were popping again.

CHRISTMAS PUDDING

As we enjoyed our Yuletide feast at the end of yet another year, I pondered on its finale. There always seemed to me a certain irony that Christmas dinner should consist of a starter, then a fattened, seasoned bird with all the trimmings and when true satiation seems to have been significantly exceeded, a flaming great pudding lands on the table.

To the Moody clan this dark, rich dessert is an age-old tradition. Stir-up Sunday was always the last Sabbath before advent when each member took their turn to make an unspoken wish while taking a stir with a big wooden spoon (being scolded for taking a lick in between!) Mother Moody ensured there were thirteen separate ingredients (representing Christ and his apostles) though father, thinking he was unseen, always added some of his own Holy spirits.

The Christmas pud as we know it, like so much else of our "traditional" Christmas, comes from Victorian times with more than a little German influence; through Albert, the Prince Consort. There is little doubt though that there were much earlier mid-winter puddings from Medieval or even pagan times. Before the days of refrigeration, making a steamed pudding was a means of preserving meat. Veal, chicken and mutton would be placed in a bag along with dried fruits and nuts which would act as preservatives, or at least partially disguise the stench and taste of crawling, rotting meat. Mincemeat was indeed meat, rather than the sweet pie-filler and delicacy that it is today.

I don't think I was ever the recipient of the famous sixpence. I recall Grandpa's denture fragmentation on one occasion and never felt it particularly worth such discomfort.

Christmas, of course, has only been celebrated in the fashion it now is, in recent years. We used to work on the day itself and it was New Year's day in Scotland that was the real holiday and festival. In the more frugal post-war days of rationing, Christmas dinner really was a feast to look forward to. Now, it seems to be yet another opportunity for general over-indulgence.

One or two of my diabetic patients asked last week if they could indulge in a wedge of Christmas pudding. After discovering that they were not surreptitiously seeking an invitation to chez Moody and with seasonal goodwill, I nodded assent. There is no such thing as a diabetic diet. Certainly one is encouraged to stick rigidly to a low-sugar and low-fat diet but as this is entirely in keeping with a healthy diet, like the rest of us they should celebrate, even indulge, but in moderation and on occasion.

"I'm sorry Mrs Moody, it was a truly fine meal and you know how I love your Christmas puddings, but just this year I thought I'd sit it out. Whether it was the extra helping of curried parsnips or the ladle-full of bread sauce, I felt I really couldn't face a dollop, with or without brandy butter. One ram's horn button from my waistcoat popped off after my second helping of goose. If I could have reached for it on the floor I would have done but I think the dog got it. I know it was a first in our household for some Christmas pud to be left but I'll take it to work in a tin for lunch through the week. Rude? Am I? Well look, I had a bowl of sherry trifle, didn't I?"

I expect she'll be talking to me again by Easter.

BLINDED

It was the twelfth day of Christmas. We may not have catered for a dozen bounding peers of the realm over the festive period, but the general disarray in the Moody household might have suggested otherwise. I don't think it was out of a sense of superstition, early that cold January morning, that I felt compelled to rid the lounge of its 8 foot decaying fir tree, now looking a little sad, stripped of its baubles and lights.

I uprooted the conical evergreen and carried it by the trunk, at arm's length. Lifting it towards the door, it caught the suspended, central ceiling light causing it to swing wildly. Fearing I would be crowned by the cast iron Victorian pendant, I glanced up, only to receive a sharp jab of twig and needles in the right eye. "Oouch" I yelled forcefully, as I determinedly dragged my assailant, blindly, to the door to cast it outside with all the force I could muster.

I returned to a sofa and sat there clutching my face, wondering if the fluid I could feel trickling down my cheek was blood or tears. I didn't dare open the eye as the pain with it shut was about as much as I could bear. How could I see my morning patients, who were perhaps already arriving, when I couldn't even see my own face in the mirror? I did what I hate most and telephoned the surgery to offer my apologies. I'd come off second best to a rogue arboreal intruder who, after a tussle, was now safely expelled from the house. My colleagues would be all the more beleaguered and probably bemused at the news. Mrs Moody descended the stairs to enquire about the commotion and the absence of her customary brew.

With no tea there would be no sympathy. Why had I tried to move the tree so hastily, before work, and would I not just look at the mess of scattered pine needles? Had I the visual acuity to have made out a single needle or even the colour green, I would have rejoiced and found a suitably witty retort.

When an eye is damaged the ciliary muscles suspending the lens often go into spasm. Even if the undamaged eye is opened to light, both pupils constrict causing pain, or literally, hatred of the light–photophobia. I asked Mrs Moody to retrieve my medical bag and we located a good mydriatic eye drop (to dilate the pupil) and an anaesthetic drop to help the pain. Under as strong a light as I could tolerate, I inspected my eye in the shaving mirror and felt there was probably no retained or penetrating piece of vegetation taking root, in readiness for next Christmas. I spent the rest of the day in a darkened bedroom listening to the wireless. Despite an hour or two of relative improvement, I had a miserable night and on each occasion when the bathroom beckoned I had to feel my way along walls and step clumsily over sleeping animals and other objects. By the following morning, the only thing that was evident was that I still could not return to work.

I was starting to lose confidence that this injury would simply repair. I felt the damage ought to be assessed by a specialist and I could think of none better that an old colleague at the infirmary. My beloved spouse agreed to cancel her hair appointment and drove me to the Eye Clinic. There, he confidently diagnosed a large corneal abrasion, or scratching of the surface of the eye, and a few marks within the anterior chamber but nothing that would not heal itself. He recommended only that I change the particular antibiotic drop I had selected. I was of course enormously relieved but didn't tell him I had an overnight bag in the car, in case he had wished to admit me to the ward. The reassurance of his words was enormous. We spoke distractedly about life and asked after our respective families. I expressed my thanks to him for running late with his lunch, or had he sandwiched me between other patients?

It was a humbling experience during these couple of days. I rushed to do a job that should have been left until a more opportune time. I had suffered from a lack of sight for a short period but long enough to be reminded how many others have to go through life. I should have sought expert advice and not stubbornly self-medicated and self-examined. I had sat on the patient's seat for once and briefly felt the uncertainty and anxieties of the feared and the unknown. Perhaps most importantly, I was reminded that in this country we have ready access to quality medical care. Yes, I had called upon a friend and could be criticized for asking a professional favour but I do know how good and available are our country's emergency services.

Three days later, I was down on hands and knees picking out every last needle from the carpet. I can say for certainty, though, that it'll be an artificial one next Christmas: a tree that is, not an eyeball.

LUNCH ON THE BEACH

The extended family were staying with us for a week. Tempers and the usual good humour were starting to wear a little thin. It was a fine spring morning and I had taken the day off work. We discussed out itinerary over breakfast and planned to head for the coast. In years gone by we would have trotted down to the station and travelled north-east by steam but sadly the facility, from here, is no longer available. Instead, we packed the cars to the gunnels and motored to the fine seaside town of North Berwick. Occasionally, one can be unlucky and have trouble seeing beyond the beach. This time there was no sea haar and the great volcanic plug of Bass Rock, that sits a mile from shore, seemed within touching distance.

We strolled along the East Sands as the children explored the rocks; finding golfballs, hermit crabs and other "treasure." We admired the Victorian architecture and Blackadder tower in the distance. It has long been my desire to have a flat in North Berwick. A beachside bolthole would undoubtedly be put to good use by family and friends. As property prices rival those of the capital though, I suspect this luxury will always elude us. Hypothetically speaking and as attractive as it would be, I would not purchase on the seafront. I fear the same climate change that enables us to picnic in early spring will also cause sea levels to rise to the point where flooding of coastal areas becomes a significant problem. This will be beyond my lifetime but, when I am six feet under, I hope any property passed on will not be submerged to a similar depth.

I was brought back to the present abruptly with cries of "I'm hungry" and "When's lunch?" We returned to the cars for trestle tables, chairs, canvas windbreaks and the carefully packed wicker hampers. The paraphernalia was assembled and the tables laid with a level of care to which even a Victorian luncheon party would have approved.

Suddenly, somebody noticed that one of the group was missing. We counted and recounted the elderly and the children, realizing wee Ernie Moody was absent. In his five short years he has always been content with his own company and imagination. He can concentrate on the game in hand (usually electronic!) with extraordinary intensity.

We called. We bellowed. We trotted up and down the beach, getting a little more concerned as each minute passed and as each call went unanswered. Eventually, Ernie was discovered crouching by a rock pool, earnestly watching the miniature sea life. Cries of relief and sharp words of reprimand followed but Ernie wondered what all the fuss was about. He knew where he had been the whole time. We headed back to our carefully prepared, but recently neglected, feast only to discover two dogs polishing off the last of it (even the Camembert and Stilton!) What had not been entirely to their palates was lying scattered, gathering sand. Despite the clear atmospheric conditions, Mrs Moody's initial reaction might have been taken by passing ships for a foghorn. She is less of a dog lover than I, and had instantly developed a pathological hatred for the beasts and their owners. She barked at the most obvious passer-by who shrugged in startled innocence. Following on was a woman swinging two leashes. She announced "sorry folks" in a breezy fashion, suggesting she failed to appreciate the mood or gravity of the situation. She explained that darling Trixie and Dixie could be such "naughty little fellows" and it was, after all, nearly their lunchtime. Mrs Moody cared little for canine gastronomic predilections and continued her salvo towards Mrs Stoneholm (clearly not of the Barbara Woodhouse mould!)

My mistake, as I later discovered, was that I did not join in the volley of disapproval and vent my anger (or express my disdain) at the out-of-control spaniel scoffing the sandwiches or the belligerent beagle bolting the bratwursts. I had been "useless" and the mere raising of an eyebrow in "faint surprise was not exactly lending support." I promised on our wedding day to the effect that I "would always stand by" Mrs Moody. On this occasion of apparent passivity (she used a stronger term!) she was less than impressed with me for doing just that. In truth, I felt the negligent, perhaps ignorant, dog walker was having the message spelled out clearly and further reiteration may have only inflamed the situation. Besides, I try not to shout at women, rather let myself be shouted at!

As a dejected and famished family group we shut up, packed up and trudged up the beach to the Seabird Centre. There, we had coffees and ice creams. We cut our losses and cut short the day, wearied from the exertions and exchanges.

We planned to have lunch on the beach and our lunch indeed ended up on the beach.

So much for a relaxing day trip. My medical services were not called upon once but I think I would rather have been at work.

ISLAND DOCTOR

I enjoy being a rural GP but for a year I was somewhat "remote." I do not mean that I was disconnected and aloof, at least no more than usual, but I worked as an island doctor.

Many summers ago, even before holy matrimony struck, the opportunity arose for me to leave these shores and work "overseas." Nothing particularly exotic really, just a choppy ferry journey over to a lesser known Scottish isle.

The previous incumbent doctor, Dr Dunn, had sadly descended into alcoholism. In a sense, he had not so much served the island community as been served by them. A posse from the Medical Council in London eventually got word of this (from a tourist interestingly, rather than a resident.) The pin-striped brigade arrived, sea-sick from the crossing, and ensconced themselves in the local hotel for a week to monitor his performance. They interviewed his patients and the physician himself before declaring the poor fellow, in their wisdom, unfit to continue in practice. A petition, signed by all on the island able to write, was not enough to save his slightly yellowed skin. I chanced upon the advert, on duty on a wet Sunday afternoon, and thought, why not? Why not indeed?

The island and its people were welcoming in their own way. As much as I adore the sing-song tones, I could not pretend Gaelic is my mother tongue and, as sacrilegious as it may seem, I prefer a glass of French wine to whisky. I think I was just suspiciously sober, in these days. Overlooking these shortcomings, the community gave me the benefit of initial doubt and took me to their bosom.

The surgery comprised of the ground floor of the house I had been allocated. Mrs May Tron doubled as both my landlady (a marvellous cook) and the local district nurse. Dr Dunn had apparently conducted most of his surgeries from a booth in the hotel (latterly nicknamed The Dunn Inn!) Local advice, generally, was to consult him in the morning before his liquid lunch, though he would usually be imbibing his liquid breakfast, elevenses or brunch. Whatever his failings, I did not find any evidence of malpractice or blunder and never a bad word about him was uttered. I did see one or two bairns in surgery with an uncanny resemblance to his image, but never voiced such observations.

There were around two-hundred residents on the isle, mostly of primary school age or elderly folk. High school children boarded during the week on the mainland and those not in the fishing industry sought work elsewhere. It was an awesome responsibility and privilege to have sole responsibility for the health of an island. In these days, before readily available helicopters and when gales prevented ferry transfers, I found myself removing appendices, delivering babies and performing other procedures I likely wouldn't have the chance, or the nerve, to do now.

The kirk still had a place and influence in the island community. Most met there, despite the effects of the ceilidh the night before, and it remained accepted that all trade came to a halt on the Lord's Day. Islanders are fiercely proud of their tradition and heritage but, I think, fear for the young. This generation expresses boredom and frustration at the lack of opportunity and employment and feels more isolated from "civilization" than did their fathers'. Depression, promiscuity, alcohol and now drugs are all too prevalent.

I did not set foot off the island in twelve months and was on duty for all of that time. They were a hardy people in the main (and on dry land too!) Midnight calls were always genuine and could not have waited until morning. I left the island having gained as much experience as I'd ever need for general practice. My contribution in that short time was considerably less that Dr Dunn's but I may yet be remembered by a few of the good people and I often think fondly of these wonderful days.

ALL HANDS TO THE PUMP

I had the good fortune recently to spend the day with my two young grandsons. Earlyish in the morning, we loaded the car with golf clubs and other sporting paraphernalia and I strapped the boys in the back (not under duress, you understand!) As we drove from the town, I noticed the fuel gauge to be indicating near empty and swung the jalopy into the nearest filling station. After waiting our turn, I connected the nozzle, ensuring that the correct "colour" had been selected (one learns from bitter experience!) and started to fill the commodious tank. Before I knew it, the boys had unclipped their safety belts and slipped from the car to see what Grandpa Ken was doing. Admiring their curiosity, rather than banishing them back to the car, I let them watch and question this all too regular and increasingly expensive ritual. Besides, I was keen to keep their attention rather than have them darting between other vehicles.

I explained that petrol is refined from oil and the world presently relies (rather too much) on this precious and diminishing commodity. Wars have been, and will continue to be, fought over it; even if ostensibly for nobler causes. Though most oil is drilled in the Gulf and in Russia, our own proud nation is a rich source. Given sufficient political drive, so to speak, Scotland could claim sole ownership and be a relatively wealthier place than at present. This may, however, be offset by cessation of subsidies from Westminster but the debate remains a heated one. I could see I was rapidly losing the boys' attention but fellow tank-fillers seemed to be looking our way. I was uncertain whether this was out of animosity at, or curiosity for, my simplistic but dull take on global and economic affairs. Either way, I felt it prudent to stop the oration. I'm no fount of great knowledge and I had certainly runneth over; as had the petroleum fount in my hand!

I replaced the cap and led the boys to the kiosk. After selecting newspapers, comics and the least sugary travel sweets I could see, we went to the counter to pay. The cashier, a lass little older than Master Moody Snr at my side, asked if I did not know that "bairns are not allowed to watch as vehicles are filled with fuel." I confessed I did not, but declared that I diligently ignore my mobile, should it ring as I replenish the combusted gasoline. Ignoring my rather irrelevant reply, she repeated and quoted as law, the breaking of which naturally invites prosecution: "Children have to remain in the car at all times." Contrary to my unsolicited pump-side wisdom, the boys interest was now at its greatest; perhaps they were just amused to see Grandpa getting a telling-off, and from someone of their own generation no less. I remained friendly but wondered, if accurate, was this not just Health & Safety forbidding yet another simple childhood curiosity? "Spillages. Petrol could get over them and cause nasty burns and allergics (sic) or even get you blinded in one eye." I could not deny these as possibilities but contended much less likely to occur when one's eager charges are standing well back. I admitted to having seen signs elsewhere about minimum purchases and advice about under-16s not using the pumps. But the diminutive observers had not been doing this, nor would I have encouraged their assistance.

The other key-clutching motorists in the lengthening queue were either faintly embarrassed (for or at me!) or demonstrated admirable patience at the old duffer up ahead. Perhaps they too were learning the laws of the forecourt.

I did not further demonstrate my age by reminiscing upon the days when her predecessor would have kindly taken the nozzle for me and chatted amicably as the numerals slowly clicked around. Now, only the most rural service stations have a cap-wearing attendant who pops from the cabin to offer such a service. These days, the digits on the dials whirl at such a rate I no longer blame my eyes for failing to keep up. I proffered an apology to "the nice, helpful lady" for my apparent ignorance of basic, modern safety issues; and me "a doctor too!"

We returned to the car, suitably educated (and I, lightly chastised.) Had Grandpa really erred in a legal or even a moral sense? (Perhaps readers could politely inform him!)

We pulled out, back onto the main road, and motored down to the golf course. The boys were quickly engrossed in tales of superheroes and Grandpa mused on whether he had subjected his grandkids to unnecessary risk.

I certainly ensured they stood well back from the swinging clubs as we each drove off from the first tee.

LICENCE TO ...WHAT?

Bond placed the receiver gently back in the cradle. The coded message had been brief but clear, it was time to go. He could not fail on this mission. He knew he was expendable but countless others depended on him. Bond had never met PC but always felt his presence and knew his licence could be revoked at any time. He reached inside his grey worsted jacket pocket for his silver cigarette holder, a gift from a Russian former lover, Vonda Dantz (codename VD). The indentation on the front was a visible reminder it had saved his life from an assassin's bullet, in Berlin two years ago. The case was all he had left to remember the girl, that and the letter from the STD people. Bond flicked it open. It was empty, of course, and he glanced at the obligatory No Smoking sign, to the right of the painting of Her Majesty. He cursed in fluent Chechen.

Bond gathered his possessions hurriedly. He would be spirited out of the country the next morning, but he had better let his landlady know as she might worry. He would have flown tonight but The European Working Time Directive 1993 forbade. He had started duty over 10 hours ago; it felt like no time at all. Before dawn he would steal out of Horseferry Road and cycle to the airport, having now attained his cycling proficiency certificate. MI5 prided itself on being the most carbon neutral secret service in post-Cold War Europe, after all. If he survived, they would frown at his report when it was noticed he had flown and not travelled by ferry and train. He meticulously rehearsed his argument but knew they disliked confrontation.

He felt instinctively for the reassuring shape of the Walther PPK. His friend; more faithful than any woman he had loved and as reliable as any fellow agent. Annoyingly, HSE disallowed him from carrying it while loaded. Bond had tried to argue this but the reply was always the same: "Health and Safety. Health and Safety." He cursed again, in passable Manadarin.

The next morning, Bond sat comfortably after strapping himself in, as the plane ascended. Did he really have to listen to the emergency evacuation details every time on these missions? It seemed hardly necessary after all his training. He didn't mind on this occasion as one of the stewardesses reminded him of a certain lady back at HQ. His feelings about Ms Moneypenny were mixed. Things had not been the same between them since she filed that complaint against him for harassment. He now knew he could not ask if she was married and his pat, after all, had only been one of affection. Sometimes Bond felt he was from a different age. He signalled to order a Vodka–Martini. He would have no choice whether it was shaken or not as the tannoy introduced the pilot as a partially-sighted double amputee, there by virtue of the Equal Opportunities programme. But Bond remembered he had to decline alcohol on the advice of his doctor. He obligingly reciprocated the steward's pleasant smile. He cursed again, in perfect Swahili.

He must focus on the mission ahead. After disembarking safely, he would be deposited a few miles from the secretive island of Crab Key. Parachutes were banned, unless of a highly luminescent yellow, for maximum visibility. This, to Bond, seemed incongruous on an intelligence gathering operation but he knew MI5's mission statement (disclosed to all those who ask, under the Freedom of Information Act 2000) and he was obliged to chant it each day. The mysterious Dr No, through a certain tax loophole which the government seemed in no hurry to close, lived there in exile. When preparing for this mission, Bond had mistakenly referred to Dr No as a "villain" but had been advised this was derogatory and discriminatory and possibly prejudicial to any future trial. The department psychologists suggested Dr No was perhaps merely misunderstood and any perceived failings were only the result of unfortunate parenting.

The grainy spy satellite photographs of Dr No's alleged missile sites, on the west side of the island, might be dismissed in court as an invasion of one's privacy. Previous pictures had apparently shown no signs of these tubular structures. Comparisons, however, could not be made as the original pictures had been destroyed under the Data Protection Act 1998. Anyway, these new images could represent Dr No's own sanitation plant, so wealthy was the man and so troubled by an inflammatory bowel condition.

Bond sat back, deciding to leave, for now, the reams of small print to be read and the disclaimers to be signed before the mission could legally begin. He closed his eyes and listened to the hum of the engines and the screams of the children, sharing Economy Class with him. He cursed yet again, in English. Would he ever be allowed to do his job properly?

1948

I'm not sure one can describe a year as good or as bad, unless perhaps if talking about wine. I think though that one can legitimately suggest one year is more significant than another in national or international terms but would have to be ready to qualify such proclamations. The year I bring to your attention might be thought of as only three years after the ending of hostilities and when rationing was still the norm. There is far more, however, to 1948 than that. Let us have a look at the events and the people in the process of turning 60.

Lulu, Walter Smith and Alexander McCall Smith would seem to be the best known Scots born that year but so was the Duke of Rothesay (HRH The Prince of Wales.) The Australian sweetheart Olivia Newton John and the, rather less attractive, rockers Alice Cooper, Robert Plant and Ozzy Osbourne also ventilated their lungs for the first time. Those who had made their marks but were taking their last breaths included: Mahatma Ghandi, Unity Mitford, Babe Ruth and Orville Wright.

On the world stage, Harry Truman was US president, Clement Attlee was prime minister and Arthur Woodburn, Secretary of State for Scotland. The United Nations established the World Health Organization and adopted the Universal Declaration of Human Rights.

In a retrograde step, Malan became president of South Africa, thus beginning the apartheid regime.

For me, 1948 was particularly significant for two reasons. Firstly, it was the year the Morris Minor was officially launched. The

"Moggie or "jelly mould" beloved by so many was the car that really brought motoring to the working classes. It was pitched at a suitable price, was roomy and was said to have superior cornering and handling. It may only have been one in a line of Morrises (between the Morris Eight and Morris 1100) made in Cowley, Oxfordshire, but by 1961 was the first British million-seller. Critics may argue this spelled the end of the traditional railway network and paved the way to traffic congestion and this may be true, but never could it have been done with such character or in greater style. I recall our family's first car, a beige Moggie complete with trafficators and two-piece split windscreen. The Morris Traveller which I bought soon after our marriage remains my favourite car and I still see it occasionally, out and about. It almost brings a tear to my eye that I parted with her (the Morris, not Mrs Moody-she's still here!)

Of only marginally less impact in my (working) life was the introduction, that same year, of The National Health Service. 1948 was in fact over 230 years after John Bellers first proposed a plan for such a service but good old Nye Bevin is the chap credited with this major achievement. Doctors are grateful for this political initiative but rightly remain sceptical and fearful of the intentions, motives and foresight (or lack thereof) of successive governments.

The NHS may indeed be "the envy of the world" and its founding principles remain largely intact: a universal service, funded by taxes, which provides care on the basis of need, not on capacity to pay. Alternatives to this, as seen in other countries, are almost too awful to contemplate. The problem is, the NHS was conceived in the belief that major disease would be eradicated and its role would be largely preventative rather than curative. Latterly, sophisticated investigations, drug costs, and the increasing tendency to over investigate in a defensive fashion have led to an explosion in the budgetary requirements. It is also, to an extent, a victim of its own success, as the increasing elderly population need ongoing care on a scale that could never have been anticipated.

The NHS is the country's single biggest employer and it is my belief, as sad as it is to say, that I do not see it being able to continue in its present "A&E"– Always and Everyone form. I suspect rationing, as was already present in 1948 albeit in a different form, will become ever more apparent. The crucial element is that this is determined by evidence and research and not left to politicians or policy-makers to decide. I also expect an insurance system of sorts to be introduced, similar to what operates in the private sector at present. The obvious problem with this is that there will be those who cannot get sufficient cover and will be denied essential or emergency care. That will be a tragedy.

The Morris Minor and the NHS are my favourite "machines" and institutions, co-incidentally created the same year. 1948 is also a significant year for this old scribe – but I couldn't possibly tell you why!

SMILE

There was a break between patients so I sloped off to boil the kettle. As I strode down the corridor, Mrs Mona Lotte our practice manager, looked at me oddly before stating that she gets worried if she sees me smiling. "Something must be wrong," she declared. Is the involuntary, and apparently rare, raising of the corners of my mouth really worthy of such comment, let alone suspicion? She muttered something about me being Moody by name and something else but I didn't quite catch what she said, as she marched off shaking her head.

I don't suppose a smile does come particularly easily to my lips. There is a cliché about fewer muscles being called into action to smile than to frown. I've never counted them, but admit I'm probably more accustomed to the latter action and reflex.

As a doctor, I would certainly be viewed with suspicion, if not contempt, were I to have a permanent smirk across my jowly chops. It would be inappropriate to grin my way through a consultation, as my patient wept into a hankie recounting her story of tragedy and loss.

I have read books written by doctors and psychologists, who claim to be in the know, that body language is an important element in any consultation or meeting. Eye contact and a warm handshake and smile apparently inspire confidence and suggest sincerity, thereby putting a patient at his ease.

Of course, a smile may not be welcoming or sincere. The fake smile of a conman, the menacing smile of an assailant, the nervous smile of an exam candidate and the grimace of someone in pain betray emotions of anything other than warmth and wellbeing. One's eyes are often the giveaway. The French neurologist, Duchenne, more famous for his pioneering work into muscular dystrophy, managed to demonstrate that genuine smiles involve muscle groups around the mouth and the eyes. Quite how the good doctor demonstrated pleasure or otherwise by applying electrical probes to the faces of "volunteers", I'll never know.

Some people sadly, as it were, simply cannot smile. One of the features of Parkinson's disease is the loss of facial expression. The rather mask-like appearance, when coupled with the typical quiet, monotonous speech can make it difficult to be understood and may wrongly imply disinterest. Others may be embarrassed about the state of their dentition, either fearful of displaying rotting teeth and gums or worried their ill-fitting falsers may be ejected. Depression is not associated with smiling and laughter but most sufferers will still have moments of light-heartedness. So-called laughter therapy has always stuck me as being a little artificial and hollow but, if people feel better after sessions of rib-tickling, good luck to them. At the other extreme, risus sardonicus is a terminal event in cases of tetanus or strychnine poisoning. Fortunately, this unremitting and untreatable intense muscular spasm features more commonly in detective novels than in British medical practice.

People with ready smiles are usually a healthier and happier bunch. I think they probably look younger too, when not feeling the weight of the world upon the shoulders. They are also treated more positively and enthusiastically by those they meet.

Well, I'm not going to sleep with a coat-hanger in my mouth or a banana placed sideways, as has been suggested. Each morning I will peer through rheumy eyes into the shaving mirror. I will hum Nat King Cole's memorable song and, using my index fingers if necessary, will reverse the shape of my mouth to get the process over with for another day.

But seriously, if that is not a contradiction, it can be too easy for the smile to be wiped off our faces, being replaced by grim, slightly hostile, looks. We may display our every emotion and happiness hardly ever features.

As painful and difficult as it will be, Mona, I'll try to look a bit more cheerful, even on these busier days. And who knows, it might be catching. Smiling and laughter are the only infectious conditions welcomed in the surgery.

A GOOD WALK SPOILED

When I first applied for the position of partner here, in what was then a sleepy rural spot, the mention of golf at lunchtimes sounded most attractive. My predecessors, now striding the perfect fairways elsewhere, described their typical working day – and how they managed to fit in a few patients as well! One colleague, Dr Albie T. Ross, indeed lived for the game and some of his patients, when feeling under par, knew to catch him at the ninth green (remarkably close to the surgery) but only after he had putted out. If they missed him there or he was in a bad mood having three-putted, he could always be found in the clubhouse from 3 o'clock onwards.

Rather sadly, "working" days of such leisure are no longer on the (score)cards. Patients have different expectations and demands of their doctors and if we are not listening to chests or tales of woe, examining lumps or visiting folk in the community then there will be dozens of insurance or other forms waiting to be completed.

My love of golf started when I was in single-figures (age, not handicap, for I never quite realized that ambition!) I used to visit my great-uncle Fred in the west coast seaside town of Largs. He and his pal, another Fred as it happened, used to take me around the fine, but hilly, Routenburn course. I recall sheep wandering aimlessly before being sent packing with a topped or sliced 5-iron, driven into the wind.

I was often challenged by these two elderly gents to earn a shilling by driving over drystane dykes. When I see the yard-high walls now I wonder how I managed to hit them so consistently. I often could only watch the ball ricochet and land somewhere behind me or deep in the gorse. Such wagers brought out the best and the worst of tempers in this budding sportsman, many decades ago.

He never joined our golfing party but I believe it was the old wag himself, Mark Twain, who described the great game as "a good walk spoiled." I don't know if he even ever hit a feathered ball with a hickory shafted club. He possibly did take up at least one invitation, only to find its mastery far harder than those of words. Given such an assessment, I think we should count ourselves fortunate he returned to his more famous pastime of musing about life on the Mississippi. Four miles is indeed a fine stroll but, as a beginner, you can often double that distance by double backing on yourself in search of wayward balls and taking the circuitous route to the green, 18 times over.

Many of my patients are at their happiest when pulling a cart with 14 sticks and chasing the dream of a perfect round. I admire players who play week in, week out and head for the sandier, coastal courses during the winter. More serious types turn up their noses at our local course and sometimes invite me to the challenges of their own which, naturally, is the finest and toughest in the county. I sometimes accept these kind offers, unless I suspect it is an excuse to pin me down at the 19th hole with a barrage of questions, best asked in the surgery.

Scotland is generally considered to be where a shepherd first struck a stone with his crook and proceeded to get it down the nearest rabbit hole: thus creating the game of "gowf." Detractors have pointed to earlier references in writings from ancient Egypt and China but it's obviously in the blood when our small nation can boast players of the calibre of Colin Montgomerie, Bernard Gallacher, Sam Torrance, Sandy Lyle, Ben Sayers, Jock Hutchison, Young and Old Tom Morris, "Gentleman" John Panton, his daughter Cathy and of course young Janice Moodie (probably no relation!)

Even though the United States has about half of the world's golf courses, Scotland has the highest proportion for its physical size and that of our population. We watch the US Masters each April on our televisions and marvel at the array of colours of the azaleas, but American golf is not how the game was conceived to be, all these years ago. Here, we do not play in predictably calm, warm and fair conditions but accept that three-and-a-half hours in waterproofs in windswept, drizzly, cold conditions on a links course in mid-July is how the glorious game was meant to be played!

When we come to expect bad weather it is all the more rewarding to be blessed with the opposite. One of my favourite working days is to finish afternoon surgery promptly and manage to meet my three golfing buddies on the first tee. There, we exchange pleasantries and anecdotes, playing down our excitement at the prospect of competitive matchplay-played in the very best of spirits, of course. We only rendezvous a dozen or so times each year but, when the wind dies and the setting sun is still warm enough to beat on our weathered faces, we too could be in heaven.

BETTING WITH PATIENTS

I had the occasion recently to place a bet with a patient. It was not a case of him putting on a line for me at the bookmakers nor is he a jockey by profession. In fact, I suspect Munro Cairns would not be supported by the average racehorse and even a Clydesdale would likely rather pull a plough all day long than gallop with him in the saddle for a few furlongs. Munro, now in his fifties, had a weight problem. It took him a while to recognize this but he eventually accepted that not all his clothes could have shrunk in the wash and his car seat really was pushed as far back as it would go. His blood pressure was on the rise and he was verging on the diabetic range. You could almost say it was on the cards that his obesity did not bode for a long and healthy life. He was dicing with death.

Munro claimed he ate reasonable portion sizes and cut the fat off his beef before grilling. He expressed bewilderment at his expanding girth and surprise that his bathroom scales indeed agreed with those in the surgery.

By and (sometimes very) large, one's weight is a result of calories in versus calories out. Nothing more complex than that. Food consumed should equate to the energy burned off by vigorous exercise. I tactfully expressed my doubts that, if he ate little more than fresh salad and lean meat as he claimed, he ever broke into a sweat from strenuous exertion. Pushing an electric mower over a postage stamp of a front lawn is hardly how Olympic hopefuls train.

Munro lives in the shadow of one of this area's highest hills. His house, lacking somewhat in originality but not inspiration, is called Ben Tuipharr View. The trouble is, Munro is a bit of a man-mountain himself. With this imagery in mind, I had an idea. I asked whether, despite opening his curtains to such a magnificent sight each morning, he had ever scaled the heights. He looked at me a little too long for the delivery of an honest answer, before stating that of course he had. Well, it had been just once, shortly after leaving school. A full generation ago. The challenge to him was therefore too great to miss. I offered Munro £50 if he could prove to me that he could reach the summit before he next consulted me. I felt the odds were the only slim thing in this bet. There was nothing to lose except a few pounds in the process, and they would probably not be from my pocket.

I wondered if I might be contravening some ethical code but I was not asking for money in return if he failed. I was only offering him the price of a pair of good hiking boots, a sense of achievement and the possibility of a healthier and longer life.

The government, after all, is considering paying smokers to give up their unhealthy habits, so how did my wager differ from that? Most gyms take care to offer those unaccustomed to exercise a graded introductory programme. Was I putting this man, my patient, at unnecessary risk of a heart attack or collapse? I certainly didn't want to read in the newspapers of a large body being carted off the hill under the headline: "Local GP and gambler orders man to march to his death."

My fears were unfounded as Munro returned a month or two later proudly carrying a photograph of himself clutching, against the stiff wind, a copy of a daily newspaper. Like a kidnap victim, the date could not be disputed, nor the sense of achievement in his grin. Furthermore, he informed me he had newly joined the local ramblers' association. Munro had placed a rock on the "pile of stones" at the summit and was aware that the pounds were now piling off him, for a change. He didn't exactly thank me but nodded his approval as I handed over two crisp twenties and a tenner.

I don't think I've started a precedent, at least I hope not. I don't really expect my salary to disappear in lost bets, along with the taxes that already consume much of it, though my patients might be the better for it. If readers were, as a result of learning this, to approach their own GPs asking for similar physical challenges I suspect they would be told to take a hike (and not with any financial incentive to do so!)

It was an opportunity, it was a wager, I took it but I doubt I really lost.

PART 2

MEDICAL CORRESPONDENCE

A SCHOOL ESSAY

I was up in our attic recently and chanced upon an old Ceylon tea chest. In it was assembled junk from over the years but one thing in particular drew my attention: an old school jotter. I sat myself down and smiled as I read my "News Pages" and early view of the world. One essay that had been set by a master might be of interest to you and, after a little persuasion from Mrs Moody, I offer it now for wider perusal for the first time in over half a century. Note the earnestness, innocence and expectations of this little chap. The following is the essay exactly as written by Master Kenilworth B Moody.

'If I was to write in no less than 700 hundred words what I want to be when I grow up and why, it would be this. I would like to be doctor of medicine who uses a stethyscope and other insteriments. This is not just because Father is a doctor or because people here and in faraway lands, such as darkest Africa where Dr Livingstone made his fabulous expeditions, always need help with their diseases but because I think I have a thing called vocation. (I used to think this was like a holiday but Mr Mortar in the lower form corrected my previous vowel error.) Being a doctor can win you a No Bell prize if you discover something a bit better that will change the whole world. These medicines called antibiotics were discovered by Dr Fleming, also a Scot, on a piece of mouldy bread and I think that cannot be very difficult if things lying around people's kitchen floors hold such wonderful antidotes to horrible diseases like galloping consumption. I once rescued a blackbird that had broken its left leg flying into our summerhouse (the doors were shut at the

time.) I splintered it up nicely but the bird died the next day. The veteran surgeon said it probably died of fright but I did a splendid job anyway. I have also heard about a man called Dr Alfred Kinsey from America. Father and Mother have his new book called the something behavior of the human male and female. (I don't know what the something word is exactly but it sounds like sacks full – but I know it has nothing to do with coal.) Father says I'll find out when I am eighteen years old or more and definitely at medical school up in the city. They seem to read this book quite a lot but when I ask to look at it they say it is not for my tender eyes and mind. I know it is about Biology and stuff and even heard from Know-it-all Young that we couldn't have been delivered by storks as the climate here is not suitable for these birds of the Ciconiiformes family and anyway I weighed over eight pounds and was born in this very house. I also want to be a doctor because I don't want to be other things like a train driver, a schoolmaster (especially Latin) or a singer like Buddy Holly. The lady behind me in church on Sunday nudged me hard when I sang "That'll be the Day" rather than "The day thou gavest Lord is ended." Mother didn't see the joke either and banned me from playing bagatelle or listening to the wireless for a whole week, so that put me off Mr Holly a bit. I don't even really want to be the first man on the moon either because everyone will be able to go their for there holidays in about twenty years time. I also like the sound of this new National Health Service too. Father says Mr Bevan is a bit of an idealist (and he does have a good list of ideas) but he thinks the system is pretty good so far. It means the poor folk can see a doctor and not feel guilty about not having enough pounds or shillings to pay for their medicines, tonics and bandages. I like the sound of deserving souls getting the treatment they need and I would like to be part of that new Service when I am able.

For all of these reasons and much more I really want to be a doctor. The End.

THE ORGAN TRILOGY

It had been my plan for a decade or more to make a lasting and notable contribution to the medical literature. I have been writing these articles for many years and the fun never wavered; but it is not these mildly humorous words I had in mind. Late in the evening, after completing my light-hearted weekly column, I straightened my tie, adopted a more upright posture and returned to my academic work. The research has been at some financial cost but also at the expense of my time and, as you are about to learn, perhaps of my reputation too. After the exhaustive text and painstakingly detailed illustrations were finally completed, I sent the manuscript, expectantly, to all suitable publishers; medical, academic and commercial. Their responses could have been somewhat more encouraging and today I received my final letter of rejection. Some dismissals were even rather polite.

The book was to have been entitled *Moody's Morbid Anatomy*; subtitle: *The Organ Trilogy*, but the gist of many rejections was that having both the words "moody" and "morbid" in the title was too negative and wouldn't even appeal to the Horror market. My alternative suggestion of "Dr Ken's Study of Solid Organs," was considered "lightweight," paradoxically, and even "lowbrow" (whatever that means.) My hopes were temporarily raised when one publisher expressed interest until he realised *The Organ Trilogy* had nothing in fact to do with Bach, Baroque or indeed anything musical. I had some sympathy with a reviewer who suggested that the study of individual organs is "old fashioned," as the modern approach is to view Anatomy as one "systemic, functioning continuum." I was a little hurt though by one wag who compared my proposals to "what is already seen on most school library shelves, and even then from generations gone by."

My cardinal mistake, in retrospect, was to have twenty-thousand dust jackets printed, before securing a publishing contract. It was only when they were delivered to the surgery that a trainee nurse pointed out that, counting the liver, pancreas, spleen and kidneys, there are actually five solid organs in the average abdomen. I would still be prepared to argue that separate chapters for the left and right kidneys are not strictly necessary but I now accept the need to "drop" an organ to ensure a trilogy does not make for the most credible or comprehensive of medical tomes. A colleague cast further doubt upon the definition of an organ and what indeed constitutes a gland or viscera.

My last ditch attempt to put the book between these dust jackets (by now truly dusty!) was with a notion to borrow Douglas Adam's concept of "A Trilogy in Four Parts." I was soon advised that my entry to the higher echelons of medical education could not be guaranteed with such a subtitle.

I now realise my work will never supersede Gray's Anatomy (I'm still waiting for the more definitive Black and White's Anatomy!) If I ever rise from the ashes of this failure, I may share with you my interpretations and insights; drawings and diagrams of our sub-diaphragmatic innards. If the editor were ever to permit such publication and just one reader learnt a single fact about their internal organs, I would count my hours of work by candlelight, while Mrs Moody pleaded with me to retire, as well spent. If these chapters were to be well received it might generate a groundswell of opinion and the publishing world may take notice and be obliged to review its previous verdict. Perhaps then my contribution to Anatomy will be somewhere between Dr Gray and Messrs Burke and Hare.

Even if this pipe dream were to come to pass, as hard as it is for me to admit, I doubt The Organ Trilogy in any format will ever be on essential reading lists or grace the shelves in esteemed seats of learning such as Harvard, St Andrews, Oxford and Galashiels.

GREETINGS FROM CANADA

During the month of December, like most other people I suspect, Mrs Moody and I enjoy opening our Christmas cards. We derive pleasure from remembering old friends; sharing in their joy at new life and in their sadness at the passing of others. Some carefully chosen and cleverly worded cards make me howl with laughter, others are no more than mere formalities. Normally, I rather enjoy studying the photographs of happy family groups and reading the enclosed newsletters. As much as I'm keen to share in the growth and progress of families, there is one card that arrives each Christmas time that somewhat raises the hairs on the back of my neck. This may seem a little ungracious and unkind. A former medical school colleague who emigrated to Canada, for some reason sees it as his annual duty to inform me of his wonderfully successful and happy family. I would probably share with him in this joy if he did not appear to rub my nose in their successes or if he expressed even a modicum of interest in my own kin. The following newsletter duly arrived by airmail this very week:

Greetings Ken and Mrs Moody. Wow, what another hectic and fabulous year the Beturov clan has enjoyed again. It's funny isn't it how I still write "clan" when we left Scotland for far better things many years ago. I guess Scotland is a good place to come from but not to end up, ay buddy? You'll want to know about us, so let's start with the children. Mitch is following in his dad's deep and successful footprints (in the snow, haw, haw!) We have no doubt that he will be awarded his professorship in Internal Medicine this year at the

National University. His adorable wife (a former Miss Canada), gave us a beautiful grandchild earlier in the year. Our second son, Weir, has become All Canada national debating champion having demolished the competition with his motion "This house believes it is far preferable to dwell and thrive here in the New World rather than exist in small, overpopulated, polluted Western Europe."

Myles, our third, meanwhile has been selected from thousands to lead the Queen Elizabeth rainforest expedition to Venezuela. The president himself will be awarding the medal of honor and we shall be dining privately with him in his residence. We find ourselves these days having less time to go on vacation for relaxation as our children's award ceremonies and graduations are, dare we say, becoming quite common! I recall you have kids Ken (can't remember their names) but suspect, like their dad, they are doing OK but not achievers in any particular sense of the word.

We moved to an even bigger house this year. We found ten bedrooms hardly enough for entertaining our legions of friends from neighbouring provinces. They usually come in the hunting season and agree that our 10,000 acres of forest and valley is probably Canada's finest for big game and fish. Weir shot his first Grizzly this fall. The beast came at him, out of nowhere. Being the best shot this side of the Mackenzie River, he hit him right between the eyes. We had the monster skinned, gutted and on the barbecue before nightfall.

Say, do you still write that silly wee column, Ken? You did have quite a good sense of humor but you'll likely have run out of interesting things to say by now. I remember when we came to stay in your small house you told some neat stories round the fire but would go all silent when I told much funnier ones and informed you how much better life and medical practice is over here. If your handful of readers have tired of your jottings, feel free to speak to your editor and, for a few thousand dollars a week, I could tell them about the wonderful life of a Canadian country physician. I never understood, Ken, why you declined our invitations to leave that small, grey, wet country for the cleaner air and healthier lifestyle of North America.

If you really do still see over forty patients every day for the meagre pay check that you do, tough luck buddy. I cruise out in the Dodge pickup to settlements, see a dozen folks, max, and send the tab to Medicare insurance. The money just rolls in. If I haven't caught a whopper of a fish for supper, I'll stop at the store on the way home for half-pound sirloins at two-dollars a piece. Beats haggis, I'd say.

Be sure to have a swell Christmas, folks. Raise a glass of your over-priced malt to us on the big day, though we make our own luck and fortune anyway. We didn't get your newsletter in your card last year. Perhaps you Moodys haven't anything different or worthwhile to say or maybe we just tossed it on the fire. No matter. Have a happy New Year too, and I'm sure you're already looking forward to our next newsletter.

Seasons Greetings
Weir Beturov MD (Hons.)

DEAR PATIENT

I felt it necessary to write to a patient. It was done after considerable thought and discussion with colleagues. I hope it illustrates that steps sometimes have to be taken and lines drawn for the sake of both the particular doctor-patient relationship and the practice as a whole. You may be rather taken aback by my frankness but I would contend this does not spill into rudeness. The following is the letter:

Dear Miss Anne Tennsety,

Thank you for your further correspondence, received this morning. I assume the bound file I have in my hand is indeed the most recently sent but I appreciate there is quite possibly a further update winging its way to me, as I write. When I first diagnosed (or, as you argue, "stumbled upon") your condition several years ago, you told me you felt a certain satisfaction. It may have been the case that other doctors missed the "obvious" signs and "neglected" to perform the necessary tests, as you allege, but I maintain that your numerous physical complaints merely manifested themselves at the time you consulted me. For this reason, I took (and was given) no credit but was pleased for you to have some sort of an answer.

You took the news of your diagnosis with a doggedness I cannot recall seeing in all my years in general practice. As I said at the time, I did not think it necessary for you to resign from your perfectly good job or terminate friendships with all but fellow sufferers. Your condition could never be considered life-threatening or even particularly serious, but I concede some changes to one's lifestyle are often indicated.

When I really felt you were taking matters rather too seriously was when you started bombarding (and I use the word advisedly) me with downloads from the online patient forums to which you subscribe. As helpful as you clearly find these to be, I confess to being rather less than convinced. It seems almost every contribution commences with a scepticial comment about the medical profession in general or certain doctors in particular. These, I have observed, border on the slanderous and would seem to be no more than unqualified, and often anonymous, opinions. I was never sure, Miss Tennsety, why you felt it necessary to include me in this correspondence. I would never expect the addressees of my letters to be receptive to the material sent if I opened with an insult. Furthermore, I did not particularly appreciate your numerous annotations, which I quote accurately: "For your necessary education, doctor" and "Pass this on immediately to your colleagues who perhaps know even less about my condition."

I carefully choose the conferences and seminars that I attend each year. I am unsure why you feel I should go to every post-graduate meeting dedicated to your condition, regardless of which end of the country it is scheduled to take place. Even if I could find the time, your travel itineraries and lists of convenient accommodation are more than sufficient, thank you. When I approached you about your, frankly overzealous, petitioning of me, you simply claimed that yours is an underdiagnosed condition in the population. This may indeed be the case, but it would be unfair to my other patients were I to spend a fraction of the time you suggest on further educating myself and evangelizing my colleagues. My own credibility might be called into question were I to take your lead and become a single-issue campaigner. You expressed surprise and dismay when I declined to supply you with details of fellow sufferers in the practice and again I cite confidentiality as just one good reason.

I confess that I have not read your increasingly lengthy epistles in quite the depth you probably believe. Perhaps, if they did not arrive on a weekly basis and were limited to, say, ten sides I may have been able to keep up. I have, however, been reading between the lines, as it were, and respectfully suggest that you may have things a little out of proportion. I sense too that you may have been testing me. You are always quick to pick up on me when

I display ignorance of the very latest research or informal correspondence on the subject from "Angry Marge in Basingstoke." In truth, I lost that particular thread some time ago.

Your copious written and printed matter remains here at the practice. We thought we were succeeding in our efforts to become a paperlight practice but instead are in discussion with joiners about having additional shelving units erected. If you could find a suitable purpose or an interested recipient we would happily arrange for vans to return the bulk of it to you, at your earliest convenience. I strongly suspect other doctors may not particularly welcome the sheer volume, but I suppose you could ask.

I know you will be disappointed by this letter and in me in general. I am sorry if I appear a little ungracious but feel, after all these years, my knowledge of your condition is adequate. I also feel we have reached a point in our professional relationship where frankness is required. I do not believe I have treated you any differently to my other patients but I fear the demands you make of me are, at best, a distraction and possibly a misuse of my time. It is to these, dare I say needier, people whom I must now turn my attention.

Yours sincerely
Dr Ken B Moody

INTERVIEW WITH DR. MOODY

Roving and intrepid journalist, Fiona Pagett, managed to track down the publicity-shy Dr Ken B Moody in his surgery last week. She gained access by wrong-footing his receptionists and got a full ten minutes of the busy medic's time. The looks from disgruntled patients and the exchange of words, for her adding to their already considerable wait, are best not described here. The following is the interview exactly as recorded:

Dr Moody, your recently published book "View from the Surgery" is already flying off the shelves. Does its popularity come as a surprise?

It certainly does, Ms Pagett. When I finally agreed for David (the book's Editor) to put together "a book" and arrange for "a book signing" I thought that was what I'd literally be doing; signing a book. I envisaged folks sharing the one volume around and it eventually being lost down the back of a sofa. I am pleased though that the publishers have a large enough printing press to cope with hundreds, or is it thousands, of copies.

I think readers would like to know if what you write is strictly accurate and the characters real patients.

Of course they are. I couldn't make up any of what I write, I just don't have that sort of imagination. Truth is stranger than fiction, I always say. I believe I once changed the name of someone to preserve her anonymity but on the whole patients love to read about themselves, or so they tell me.

Dr Ken, do you mind if I call you that? Gosh, your desk really does look like the cover of the book-just a little more cluttered. What is the significance of the red apple?

Please, call me Ken. May I call you Fiona? Well my views, as expressed within the book, are often rather black and white but the room, as you'll notice, is in fact technicolour. The apple, I think, signifies the wish for good health.

As in, an apple a day keeps the doctor away?

Perhaps, dear, but from my point of view, an apple a day keeps the patients at bay!

That's a photo of Mrs Moody on your desk, isn't it?

It is indeed a photo of Mrs Moody, but I don't think it was taken with her on the desk! Yes. Marvellous lady. She might appear a little old-fashioned, and in some ways she is, but she remains my love, my life, my soul mate. There's a whole piece dedicated to her in the book – it would come as a surprise to her if she ever read it and I don't think I'd wish to be in the same room if she did!

That's very touching. Except, perhaps, the bit about being old-fashioned. She sounds a rather special person. In just one word, how might you describe her?

Long-suffering.

But that's two words.

Oh you are pedantic! Tolerant, then!

OK, moving on. You certainly have a nice view from your surgery window, Ken. Is this an inspiration to your work and your writing?

Absolutely. My work is my writing and my writing is my work. See yon hill in the distance, I used to climb that, have my beef and mustard sandwiches at the top and be back in time for afternoon surgery.

Pretty impressive, I suppose things are just too busy nowadays to find time to do that.

No, not really. It's just that I get out of puff and have developed a touch of rheumatics.

But, are these not golf clubs I see over there in the corner? Good that you get some exercise but that seems a bit stereotyped, does it not? Doctors and golf. I would have expected a skeleton or something, standing in the shadows.

Stereotyped? Me? Never. I rarely manage to play the great game. I just didn't have enough room in the boot of my car and I have the first game of the season tonight. No, I don't have a skeleton in the surgery (or even in the closet!) but I do plan to donate my body to Medical Science, if they'll have me. Who knows, it might be more than just my spirit that lives on, here in the surgery, after I'm gone!

Yes, you're obviously no spring chicken Ken, is retirement on the cards?

Jings, you don't mince your words, Fi. But you're right, I'm nearer the evensong of my career than the dawn chorus. And these cards you refer to over there, I'll have you know, are Thank You cards from grateful patients. I don't know exactly, but while work here gives me material for the articles (and the books) I'll keep going; perhaps until the patients or the powers that be deem otherwise. Until the letters of complaint outnumber the Thank Yous.

Your weekly newspaper column has been running for a few years and remains as varied and entertaining as ever. Will there be other books in the future?

It depends. I write for the enjoyment of it. It's a release of sorts and some consultations, I feel, just have to be recorded for the benefit of others. If my jottings are studied closely and picked over there may be snippets of helpful information and advice to be found but I write in my own semi-literate way, mainly to amuse. There will never be any shortage of material with life here in the surgery, such as it is. I'll write 'til the pen runs dry or, more accurately, 'til the Corona typewriter ribbon can't be replaced. So, in answer to your question, I wouldn't be surprised if other books follow.

And are there any new ventures for "View from the Surgery"; as if the prospect of further books isn't exciting enough?

I'm a great supporter of the spoken as well as the written word. *The Talking Peeblesshire News* is the product of a worthy band of people. These good folks give freely of their time and meet regularly to record the contents of the paper for the benefit of others, unable to read it for themselves. Blindness and other visual impairments shouldn't be reasons for exclusion and I've been happy to lend a hand or (being more precise with the anatomy) my tongue, by reading some of my articles.

Has this been well received by listeners?

I'm led to believe so, lass. Both the Talking PN and the Royal National Institute for the Blind (RNIB) are interested in continuing to broadcast my scribblings. The only criticism has been that I speak too slowly! I suspect they'll get a better reader to do the job and I've no problem with that. I know nothing about gadgetry but the website that David set up (Viewfromthesurgery.com) has audio recordings on it. He says this is the way of the future and he may be right. I really must learn more about the internet but I understand the website is worth a look.

Well, that about wraps it up, Dr Ken. I think that name suits you best! It's been a real pleasure meeting you. You were a bit more forthcoming than I imagined you'd be. Thanks ever so much for seeing me today.

What, you're not here in any medical capacity then? You're not a patient?

Well no, not exactly. Not here anyway.

How on earth did you get past the fearsome receptionists then?

Journalistic experience I think you'd call it.

I see. Well it's been a wheeze!

Rather like when you now try to climb that hill out there!

That's enough, young lady! I make the jokes around here.

Anyway, would you sign my copy of 'View from the Surgery', Dr Ken.

Of course I would. Have you got a pen?

There's one on the desk.

A DOCTOR'S OCCUPATION

On our recent (and first) trip to Jersey, I found myself lacking somewhat in reading material. That was until I stumbled upon a fine little paperback. I had been curious to find out more about the German Occupation of The Channel Islands (1940-1945) and here was a book, by a GP on Jersey, during the whole of that troubled time.

A Doctor's Occupation was written by Dr John Lewis in 1982. Like so many others who survived the war, he chose not to talk about his experiences for several decades but later felt that a record should be made, for the benefit of others.

Dr Lewis hailed from Wales and trained in London. He fell in love with Ann, a girl from Jersey and, when in 1935 a vacancy for a GP partnership arose, the opportunity seemed too good to miss. Life "could not have been more wonderful," and they even honeymooned in the splendour of Crieff at £1 per day! The subsequent few years of "entertaining and being entertained" were most pleasurable and he admitted to a naivety about the storm clouds gathering over Europe.

After a turbulent period, the partnership with Dr J.J. Evans dissolved and Dr Lewis started to become aware of the very real threat posed by Hitler. Rumours emanating from Poland were that male babies were being taken from parents, for the purposes of strengthening The Reich. Up to half of all islanders made efforts to leave and, with Ann now heavily pregnant, they returned to the relative safety of Wales. This was in spite of him forfeiting all his capital to his profiteering former partner. Dr Evans had remained and agreed to look after Dr Lewis' patients and the further financial benefits of doing so would have seemed attractive. Soon afterwards however, Evans "without a word of warning and without making any arrangements for our patients, had unaccountably panicked and left the island." Dr Lewis was so concerned, particularly for his maternity patients, that he felt duty-bound to return to Jersey. Before his own first child was born, he did just that, but events took over and he found himself trapped on the island for the next five years.

Jersey and the other Channel Islands, despite Churchill's concerns, were felt to be of "little strategic importance" and became a demilitarized zone. The Germans quickly moved in by mounting air raids, killing eleven islanders, and I notice one victim was a William Moody.

Jersey and Guernsey were regarded by the occupying force as the "first stepping stone to England." They were the only part of the British Isles ever to be under German control and there was a ratio of one soldier to every four islanders. There were ten doctors for the 40,000 inhabitants. The Nazis, of course, had their own medical personnel and would not tolerate help from civilian medics, even when offered on several occasions.

Dr Lewis felt he could do nothing other than "throw myself totally into the practice."

He was aware that commodities and luxuries were becoming scarcer and so paid early visits to his tobacconist and wine merchant, buying what stock he could. I enjoyed reading the details of how he later distilled his own gin and nurtured tobacco plants. It was interesting to note some of his priorities during these times of ration, uncertainty and hardship. His prized car, however, was requisition by the Germans and he often saw it being used by officers, clearly on social rather than official business.

He was determined to keep in touch with world events and hid a wireless set in a chimney breast, despite the punishment for such being execution.

He remained a compassionate and dedicated doctor. People of course continued to suffer from usual ailments and illnesses but other needs arose. One Jewish lady, knowing she was to be deported, consulted him seeking medical exemption. He agreed to fake a major abdominal operation by creating a scar, under local anaesthetic. The lady, frustratingly, was against such disfigurement and declined.

Local girls who "made no attempts to resist the advances of German soldiers"were known as "Jerry bags." Babies were soon born as a result of these unions. The hostility towards the new mothers eventually lessened and the German authorities did not condemn what it believed was a natural part of The Fatherland taking over the world.

As the Occupation and war dragged on, food, medicines and supplies became still scarcer and the general health of the population declined. School-aged children were on average somewhat shorter than those in less troubled times and infectious diseases became more prevalent. Dr Lewis attended a 7-year old boy with advanced diphtheria and knew the antidote in his possession might be wasted on the dying lad and could be used for someone in whom there was greater hope. Thirty or so diabetic patients were admitted to hospital when insulin supplies ran out. This was to ensure a scrupulous diet with minimal exertion. Hopes were raised when a box marked "Insulin" arrived on the island but tragically it had been raided, probably in France, where conditions were thought to be even worse. All but one of these patients perished and, by cruel irony, supplies arrived days after the last one died.

Petrol rationing became so severe that Dr Lewis latterly travelled to all his daytime house visits by bicycle (inner tubes replaced with garden hosepipe!) and only night visits were by car.

Such oppressive circumstances as war and occupation bring out the very best and worst in people. The settling of old scores and bearing false witness against neighbours often had murderous consequences. People had their homes burgled, livestock stolen and vegetable patches raided. Others would put their lives at risk to hide fleeing and condemned persons, even those unknown to them.

The war did eventually come to an end. The surrender was not preceded by atrocities, for the Germans knew they would be judged on their actions.

There were many deaths of islanders during these five years, most being from deportations to camps on mainland Europe. Mrs Lewis returned to Jersey with their 5-year old son (who he only then met for the first time.) They moved to a centrally placed, more rural house and raised three further children.

Jersey was forever changed. Dr Lewis was forever changed but remained there the rest of his days.

A Doctor's Occupation
ISBN 0952565919
Dr John Lewis

IS MEDICINE A VOCATION?

It seemed to be a big blow to some of our patients when we handed over our out-of-hours responsibility to NHS 24. Since the days of yore, general practitioners practised in an "any time, anywhere and anyone" fashion. In this traditional rural, farming community, evening and night calls were usually for pretty genuine reasons and really could not have waited until morning. We were often met with profuse apologies from patients and their attentive relatives. In more recent years, sadly, our consumer rights-driven-society-with-attitude had reached even here and out-of-hours calls were demanded rather than requested. Working hours were often just "not convenient" for the busy patient.

Since making this change a few years ago, we have been on the receiving end of all sorts of criticism for "letting the side down." One patient even wrote to a national newspaper suggesting that this was the turning point and Medicine is clearly no longer a vocation, leaving only ministers of religion in this category. In case we missed his letter he sent us a copy for our information. It left me wondering: what is a vocation; did I ever have one; was this indeed the turning point and does it really matter anyway?

My well-thumbed dictionary defines "vocation" as being: "an urge, inclination or predisposition to a particular calling or career," from the Latin *vocare*: to call. Urges, inclinations and predispositions tend now to be used only with reference to one's urology or sexuality!

I suspect few doctors can honestly claim, with today's bureaucracy and the demands now upon us, that we are still pursuing our chosen "vocation." Probably the oldest cliché at a medical school interview is when a bright, earnest young thing declares that he wishes to embark on a medical career in order "to save lives." Rather than being taken as disarming honesty, it usually results in instant rejection with the cynical suggestion that he joins the Fire Service.

The three traditional vocations or professions (ignoring the proverbial oldest profession for the time being!) are the Clergy, Medicine and the Law. General practice seems to have adopted some of the Clergy's role by becoming an ear and shoulder for the depressed, the sad and the bereaved. As to whether the Law should ever have been seen as a vocation I cannot say, but some would have sympathy with Shakespeare (*Henry VI*) when he said: "The first thing we do, let's kill all the lawyers."

I don't think Medicine is a vocation any more and I am not sure that, for most doctors currently practising, it ever was. I suspect having-or being in-a vocation, to our pontificating patient, implies being caring and compassionate and putting patient before self (and family). I have yet to meet a doctor who did the latter and didn't have regrets. Our regulating body, the General Medical Council, reminds us that doctors have a "duty of care" and the majority of us try our level best, respect and are polite to our patients (even my erstwhile colleague Dr Bodie Aiken, in unguarded moments!) I believe the best I can do is to be a competent, up-to-date, non-judgemental doctor with a seasoning of friendliness and humour. To some it may sound like a minister denying the existence of God, but I confess to not practising medicine now out of a sense of vocation. Being emotionally detached, I believe, is a good thing. Furthermore, my sense of vocation such that it was, has really been weathered out of me.

It's a job and only a job, but occasionally it can be the most satisfying and rewarding one in the world.

DR KEN REPLIES

Dr Moody received a letter written in response to his article "Is Medicine a Vocation?" The following is both that letter and his considered reply.

Dear Dr Moody,

I write primarily as a doctor's daughter, but also as a retired nursing sister and midwife. Giving of my time generously in the community, I am aware of people's needs and their feelings towards the medical practice.

I read with interest your article "Is Medicine a vocation?" and sadly have to agree that it is no longer the case.

I can well understand your reasoning as to why this has come about but totally fail to understand why a GP expects his patients should be ill between the hours of nine to five from Monday to Friday, and outside these hours (comprising two thirds of the week) he/she can hand over his/her flock to an unknown voice at the end of the telephone.

My father was a GP surgeon, who practised for forty years. Bar New Year's Eve and usually two weeks annual holiday he was "on call" every night including weekends and refused point-blank to embrace exchange interception. As a family we knew that the patients came first and we never objected, felt deprived or neglected. He visited the elderly routinely and knew his patients' situations and responsibilities. To me he had a real vocation.

On retiral in 1966, he stressed "The Crying Need for Care of the Aged" and pointed out the decline of filial responsibility. He reminded the young that they too would be old one day. Forty years on, the same applies but the elderly have increased in number, filial duties have further declined and the young have less respect for the old.

In this area, so heavily weighted with elderly, many on their own, I have met genuine apprehension amongst them, particularly on a Friday night, lest they should become ill over the weekend-is this acceptable?

I wonder why, Dr Ken, the practice cannot operate some form of rota to cover off-duty hours or at least provide a live kent voice to give advice over the telephone.

We all know things have changed, Dr Ken, but why is it that with the tremendous progress technology has brought, so many folks are disillusioned? Wouldn't you agree that the pendulum has swung too far and needs addressing?

Medicine may no longer be a vocation but surely there could be real satisfaction in providing a standard of service that meets the needs of the practice's patients.

Yours sincerely,

May B Ayling

and in reply...

Dear Mrs Ayling,

Thank you for your letter and the interesting points you raise.

Your father truly was a fine man, I am sure, but I would respectfully suggest the world of 1966 bears little resemblance to that of today. The Elderly have indeed increased greatly in number, often with the attendant problems of old age. Unfortunately, the notion of "visiting the elderly routinely" is truly historical. In surgery, we can each see up to 60 patients per day and this restricts our time for home visits greatly. If we could even call upon the chronically and seriously ill routinely, this would be a attending to a more specific need. Personally, I would enjoy taking tea with older people on a regular basis but would only be further criticised by patients waiting back at surgery and probably by the GMC too!

It is not a case of "expecting" patients to be ill during surgery hours (8am to 6pm incidentally, and not "nine to five.") NHS 24 is not without its faults, but I believe the objective opinion (verbally and in person) provided by these medical and nursing colleagues is of no lesser quality and certainly not to be dismissed. We notify them of patients with certain conditions, particularly those in whom we might anticipate problems. True emergencies, as ever, are dealt with by the ambulance service.

I'm afraid I have never considered myself as having a "flock." This implies patients are passive, sheepish, lacking in responsibility and in need of constant guidance. Lack of personal responsibility is indeed the case with some people, as demonstrated in the latter years of us providing 24 hour care. Some of the reasons for night time calls were truly astounding; yes, even requests for sick lines, holiday vaccinations and enquiries about the opening times of local sports centres!

GPs are neither shepherds nor sheep. I am not aware of any other medical practices on mainland Britain that continue to provide true round-the-clock care in the fashion of your dear father's practice. This is not the reason that we too finally relinquished struggling to be everything to everyone, all of the time. We were sleep-deprived and not able to provide an adequate and safe level of care during daylight hours.

Being a "live kent" voice is one thing but any level of service has to anticipate visits to patients, 24 hours a day. This voice, through necessity, cannot be from the one person, however much a sense of vocation he or she may possess.

Yours sincerely,
Dr Ken B Moody

A WORD OF THANKS

"It's you who writes that column in the paper, isn't it Dr Ken?" enquired Ava Drider. I had to own up and admit that it is, but there's nothing really to hide is there? I have been writing these articles for several years now on all manner of subjects. As a doctor I have to be careful that confidentiality is not breached, but after ensuring that Jean McPatient will not open her copy on a Friday afternoon and recognise details known only to her and me, this sanguine doctor has a fairly broad canvas upon which to paint.

Whether the editor was just filling a pregnant pause in the consultation or genuinely had come to see me on matters journalistic I'll never know, but as he put his socks back on he asked me in his own inimitable style if I'd write a few lines each week. I confess that I had my reservations about being able to sustain a column, with my limited vernacular or write anything that would be of the slightest interest to the good folk of the Borders, but the promise of shortbread and a pint was too much to resist.

I never wanted my offerings to degenerate into an advice column. Sunday, and other, newspapers have plenty of earnest docs willing to slowly remove their spectacles, close their eyes in contemplation and offer up sage advice. Most of this advice I notice concludes with the suggestion that correspondents consult their own doctors about the given matter. So, being one of these doctors who already receives such "referrals," I am not prepared to jump on that particular medical roundabout. I think it is rather a shame that some people feel unable to discuss certain matters with their own doctor. As GPs we are undoubtedly bogged down with everyday life and work but are failing in our duty if we are not seen as approachable. I am keen that this column is a bit lighter than that though. It will never change your life, or mine, but while I don't fully concur that "laughter is the best medicine", (undoubtedly antibiotics are!) a good chortle can make life just that little more bearable or turn a bad day into a good one.

I have been truly staggered by the response I have received since starting this venture. In truth, when I invited comments I expected just the odd criticism to the effect that my facts were imperfect or that my grammar and punctuation are woeful. While this indeed may be the case, the remarks and enthusiastic support from the readership has been quite breathtaking. Okay, my chest is now somewhat more bronchitic than that of a smoking, pigeon-fancying retired miner, but you'll know what I mean. I need only check my email now and a veritable smorgasbord of anecdotes, wisecracks and inspired suggestions greet me each time. Mrs Mona Lotte, our Fuhrer of a practice manager, has noticed that I seem to have less time for coffee these days and that I have a suspiciously fixed smirk across my chops. She asked if I was having an affair, and although I did not deny it (my peccadilloes being none of her business) in a way I am. As I reply to your queries, as any good columnist must, and pen responses to suggested articles or search for evidence of your more incredible comments, I am aware my priorities are changing. My own patients come first, you must understand that, they are my bread and butter you are only my shortbread, but I write this by way of thanks and ask that you continue this most marvellous encouragement that you give me. I promise to try to honour your support, live up to your expectations and give back as good as you give.

SELLING ONE'S BOOK

As one or two readers will probably be aware, I published a book last year. *View from the Surgery* was released to varied reviews, comment and criticism (and that was just within the practice!) Most pleasingly, it was not met with indifference. I won't pretend it even reached the foothills of the national bestsellers lists but, as far as all involved were concerned, it was a sparkling success.

The best piece of advice David (the editor) and I took was to introduce ourselves to local, independent bookshops. This endangered species is an indispensable part of the promotion of a lesser known author's book. We approached our local bookshop after I was finally convinced that formally binding my boxfile of newspaper articles was better than throwing it on the fire. Some reviewers may disagree with this! Bookshop owners, who have often spent their working lives immersed in the sale of tomes of all types, informed us that a book nowadays really is judged by its cover. Browsers are unlikely to pick up a paperback if the cover image is unimaginative and uninspiring. We took a snap of my cluttered desk and it was considered a fitting eye-catcher.

I remain in touch with around a dozen of these fascinating and welcoming shops and galleries and like little better than to drop by at weekends for a blether with staff. I am tickled to hear about customers' comments and given reasons for purchase. Many people seem to have retired medics and nursing sisters in the family and express the notion that *View from the Surgery* harks back to a bygone, gentler age and would appeal to Uncle Findlay, who "always did have a wicked sense of humour."

Then there are High Street chains. Having spent time in smaller, independent bookshops, listening to the views of vendors, I garnered a certain suspicion of the larger businesses with their 70% off or "buy 7 for the price of 4" offers and their window displays featuring celebrity bestsellers. I am not in the least bit jealous, of course, that these faces of popular culture sell more copies of their autobiographies in a single week than our book will sell in a lifetime. We did a lot of legwork in the first few months. Mrs Moody and the grandchildren were often delighted at the prospect of day trips to unexplored towns and villages throughout Scotland but usually followed up their glee with a question about how much time Gramps was planning to spend "shamelessly flogging his book."

I was invited to talk about the book on the radio. These experienced interviewers put me at my ease and I was impressed by their professionalism, knowledge and interest. Despite this, I enjoyed the book signings more than any other aspect of the promotion and sales process. There is the old joke about unknown authors, where an unsigned copy of their book is rarer than a personalized one. There possibly are more copies out there with my barely legible good wishes than those without such an inscription but that, to me, is no marker of success or otherwise. I was initially reluctant to put myself forward in such a way, being concerned that I might be mistaken for a competent author or, worse, be thought to be masquerading as one. I was also mindful that my patients might think I was compromising on confidentiality but anyone who has read even some of this collection of anecdotes will know there is no fear of that whatsoever. I discovered that the quality of one's writing isn't really the point; signings are just an opportunity to meet actual and potential readers–and to discover that they do exist!

I recall one chap who sidled up to where I was sitting and expressed apparent interest in the book. He quickly brought the conversation round to his own health. Not being his doctor, I was reluctant to venture an opinion about his gastric condition and suggested his own GP's (laboriously described!) management sounded perfectly fine to me. Having received as good a "second opinion" as he was going to get he left, promising to return with the due change to purchase the book. He was never seen again. Others attended to share with me their opinions about the NHS and its perceived failings. One earnest lady took me to task for once describing teachers as stressed individuals. One must never generalize, I conceded, but I only comment upon my own observations. My favourite attendees, though, were those who dropped by to tell me they had read the column for years and wished to meet the old goat himself. I'm not sure I ever live up to expectations but, if there was disappointment, most were good at disguising it. To some, I was older than expected and, to others, younger. Some expressed an enthusiasm for my musings and admitted they now limit their reading of medical matters to me and one or two better known scribes in the weekend national newspapers.

The wheeze that we embarked upon was never going to make money or even pay for itself. Indeed, many of the book signings ran at a financial loss. This wasn't really because few copies were sold but because the overheads exceeded any profit. I am happy to take only a few shillings for each copy sold and after travel, parking tickets, wine and shortbread, my purchase of classic and contemporary fiction and gifts to the accompanying musicians, I was usually out of pocket.

So, the book continues to trickle away and I still receive lovely letters from readers around the country. Inspired by the pleasure it has been and the endless source of material from the surgery, you are now reading book number two.

PART 4

CASE STUDIES

THE SUN

I've known Saul Orr since our school days together but never really warmed to him as a person. He is bright, even brilliant, but an abrasive, over-confident sort of chap. Some say he is arrogant enough to consider himself the centre of the universe. When younger, he was a large, red-haired and undeniably handsome chap and girls used to wilt in his presence. Love rivals were often just left in the shade. Being fair-skinned though, his endless and futile pursuit of a bronze tan in the Caribbean led to him attending me again today. The years of hatless baking under a scorching sun had left his great dome of a head pockmarked and cratered, ironically rather like the surface of the moon. Multiple basal and squamous cell skin cancers have arisen and Dr Burns at the Dermatology department and myself continue to see him monthly to freeze or remove the latest suspicious lesions. His ears have been particularly badly affected and the tops were removed through necessity by the plastic surgeons. Today, as every other day and rather self-consciously, Saul has got his hat on (hooray!) but it really is a case of too little, too late. The damage has been done. Understandably, he is getting a little fed up with the never-ending need for treatment and the only solace he has is that we've never detected the worst skin cancer of all, malignant melanoma. This particularly nasty tumour is becoming ever more common. Several times each week patients present me with pigmented skin lesions and query whether they are turning malignant. It is said that only one in a million moles undergoes this change and most serious skin tumours arise from previously normal skin. Some individuals have so many moles that giving reassurance or even remembering their distribution and nature is practically impossible. For this reason, larger hospitals use digital scanning cameras and patients are invited annually for total body imaging. Computerized comparative analysis is far more efficient at detecting subtle changes than we are, and earlier intervention can occur.

The sun was considered by the ancient Greeks to be one of seven planets, hence the days of the week and their names. It is the source and sustainer of life. I do not mean this in a reverential or religious way. Some peoples, such as the Aztecs, treated it as a deity but there are still plenty of sun-worshipers in our temperate climate. On a warm summer's day our public parks and beaches are full of scantily-dressed people lying about until they are as red as lobsters. It seems, in our rather unpredictable climate, people must grab a tan when, and as fast as, they can. Ours is an image-counts-for-everything culture and glowing tans are perceived as adding to one's beauty. Dark-skinned races are spared such shallowness and are fortunate enough to be hardly ever subject to skin cancers. I get heated about very few things but I am dead against sunbeds and salons. They are highly dangerous items and facilities and are undoubtedly contributing greatly to the exponential rise in skin cancers in this country. I recall one bride-to-be who felt it necessary to top up her tan before her big day. She popped round to a salon, donned the supposedly protective goggles, stripped off and promptly fell asleep. She rather resembled a beetroot on the day, save for the two white discs for eyes. The Best Man could not resist comments about sightings of the rare but cuddly red panda. Her tears counted for little compared to the considerable damage and aging her skin had suffered.

The sun is a star, the nearest one to us, and sits at the centre of the solar system. It is composed of chiefly hydrogen and helium, so it is really gas rather than solid. It is inconceivably hot, of course, but within its structure temperatures vary some 2,000-fold. As every stargazing school pupil knows; planets, asteroids, meteorites and comets orbit the sun. Amazingly, its mass is 99.8% of the entire solar system and it is the equivalent in volume to a million Earths. At a modest 93 million miles, we are only the third closest planet, which is perhaps just as well when you consider the temperatures on the closer and more distant ones. The boffins calculate that the sun has been in existence for 4.5 billion years and has approximately the same again to go before the lights finally go out. So relatively speaking, like Saul and myself, it is somewhat middle-aged.

An excess of sun, from a health point of view, is invariably bad but in moderation is essential. Saul Orr himself would now readily agree to such moderation and the use of sun creams and protective clothing. I zapped his scalp again. He replaced his hat and touched the brim as he departed, until the next time.

HGV MOT

On busy, interminably long weekends while still a junior house doctor, I used to dream of life on the open road. I imagined days free from constant interruptions and pressures. Up there in the cab I would have time to think and listen to afternoon radio plays or lesser known piano sonatas. I would doff my cap to other kindly drivers. I might stop at chosen rural spots and drink leisurely from my flask and eat sandwiches. The anonymity and loneliness of the long-distance lorry driver seemed a desirable alternative to life on the wards. The reality is of course rather different. I never left Medicine and those who do transport freight from one end of the country to the other would scoff at such descriptions. Our congested roads are filled with car and van drivers who gesture rudely and drive dangerously. There are delivery deadlines that pay no heed to tailbacks, roadworks or closures. Being subject to satellite monitoring and speed and rest governance is probably more stressful than most other occupations. The closest I ever came to getting behind the wheel of one of these monsters of the highway was when hitch-hiking around the north of Scotland but I regularly meet these, generally amiable, drivers on a professional basis, here in the surgery.

Last week it was Harvey Lawrie who attended for his annual Heavy Goods Vehicle medical. This "MOT", as he called it, used to be the only reason he came to surgery and it was almost a mere formality, but this time it was different.

Drivers can first apply for their HGV licence on reaching the age of twenty-one. Providing they are in good health, they need not be subject to another medical examination until they reach forty-five. It is then reviewed every five years until one blows out sixty-five candles (providing the lungs still have the puff!) and annually thereafter. It is drivers in this latter group whom I get to know best. Harvey's age group is the one that presents the most challenges, from a medical point of view.

I dedicate half an hour to each of these examinations and conduct one or two each week. The DVLA has pretty clear criteria for failure. If a driver has: diabetes requiring insulin; epilepsy; poorly controlled blood pressure; a psychiatric illness; alcohol dependence or Parkinson's disease there is no issuing or renewing of the licence. It was not for either of the last two disqualifiers that Harvey was shaking slightly but for another reason. Earlier in the year he had suffered a nasty eye injury. He used to say that he had no difficulties adapting from driving a 26-ton, 4-axle vehicle to his own modest 1,100 cc. car but he had absent mindedly stooped to retrieve a dropped pen and caught the corner of the open driver's door. This penetrating injury had burst the anterior chamber of the eyeball, dislodged the lens and Harvey found himself under the surgeon's knife later the same day. The treatment reduced the pressure from the bleed but failed to repair the extensive damage. He had not needed enucleation but now, on that right side, can barely distinguish light from dark or see his hand in front of his face.

Both his Ophthalmologist and I advised him to notify the DVLA without delay. He had neglected to do so, knowing his licence would be revoked. Instead, he waited for the medical forms to drop through the door before facing the inevitable. The inevitable, of course, was that I would chide him for breaking the law these last few months, go through the motions of re-examining his vision before jotting down the numbers on the report that would bring an end to his job, income and livelihood of the last forty-five years. I had some sympathy for him but know that the rules are as they are for reasons of public safety. Even if I had wished, I could never turn a blind eye to his blind eye.

He would also be charged as usual for this, his final, HGV medical. He had hoped to drive until he was seventy, when his paltry pension for transporting poultry would have been fattened up a bit. He would have to rely on a nest egg now, if he had one.

Harvey Gaulph Victor Lawrie, as was the unabbreviated name on his passport and licence, had reached the end of the road but he did see it coming.

THE JAW

"These headaches are definitely getting worse. I've got tunnel vision and, it's maybe nothing, but my teeth just don't seem to meet the way they used to. Worst of all, my friends now call me The Jaw." My attention had indeed been drawn to Mandy Bull's oversize chin and lower face. I had not seen her for several years but sat listening intently as she catalogued her many symptoms and complaints. I was worried about the blood pressure reading I had just measured and her urine specimen suggested she may have developed diabetes. If I had not read Mandy's name on her medical records I would probably not have recognized her for she was physically quite different. Her head, though probably no larger and despite the heavy jaw, had a more prominent brow and her features seemed coarser. I examined her mouth and noted that her tongue was huge and her lower teeth projected half an inch beyond her upper incisors and canines. No wonder her speech was different, with its lisp, to the point of now being poorly understood.

From a purely professional and academic point of view, Mandy's case was fascinating; one that a doctor may never get to diagnose in a forty-year career. She was suffering from acromegaly. Derived from the Greek, the word literally means "large extremities." This condition affects about 1 in 10,000 people and most commonly presents in middle age. A growth within the pituitary gland of the brain produces a pathological excess of Growth Hormone. As the growth plates in adult bones have fused, there is no further lengthening but various "soft tissues" continue to grow abnormally.

Mandy Bull's main concern was her jaw. She felt it looked masculine and out of all proportion. My immediate concerns were less cosmetic and more for her general health. Although the tumour responsible for acromegaly is almost always benign the effects can be serious. Ultimately, and if left untreated or undiagnosed, kidney and heart failure result. I explained that she might need medication, radiation, surgery or a combination of these to deal with the underlying problem. Mandy was relieved there was an explanation and treatment for her problems but disappointed that her features would not return to their former appearance.

The jaw, or mandible, in literature has various connotations. Many heroes are described as having a jutting or "lantern" jaw; implying determination, fortitude and courage. These dashing, wholesome chaps will always prevail against adversity to win the day. Upper-class, dim-witted fools on the other hand, might be described as having recessive chins or being "chinless wonders," implying weakness or even inbreeding and the genetic consequences of that. Double-chinned characters with their extra folds of fat in the form of dewlaps are often considered to be decadent, portly or too pompous for their own good. As one ages the gums recede, the teeth become longer, decay and fall out. The jaw appears to protrude more but it is probably a relative feature. We associate hooked noses that almost meet a pointed chin with witches or Mr Punch, suggesting nastiness or malevolence.

Most problems in surgery concerning the jaw are due to pain or clicking, usually from arthritis, of the temporo-mandibular joint. The TMJ is where the mandible hinges (articulates) with the skull. Dislocation can occur, even with yawning, but more often as a result of being biffed. The mandible should always be X-rayed in such circumstances as a fracture quite possibly has also been sustained and, if so, will likely need surgical correction.

Some medical conditions, amongst other defects, cause children to have undersized jaws (micrognathia.) In extremes, there may be swallowing or breathing difficulties and the lower teeth may be bunched or awkwardly placed. Alternatively, certain facial and mouth cancers erode the mandible or their surgical treatment may result in part or all of the jaw being removed.

Mandy was seen by the endocrine and surgical specialists. Her pituitary tumour was dealt with but she was left with her mandibular disproportion (prognathism), diabetes and hypertension problems. Her self-esteem seemed to improve over the following months. She appreciated her condition was not malignant and would now not worsen. She even had the good humour to suggest that, though never a literary heroine, she had taken her condition and all that it had thrown at her squarely on the....chin.

A DEVILISH CONDITION

Yuri Kassid limped into the room and planted himself heavily onto a chair. He wore a polished brogue on his right foot and a slipper on his left. Yuri and his brother were restaurateurs and presentation counted for much. Knowing he was always immaculately attired, I had a fair idea why he should display this apparent fashion faux pas. With great deliberation and care, he removed the designer slipper, rolled down his Argyle sock and showed me a swollen foot which, as if in cartoon fashion, almost pulsated before my eyes. Gout is often a rather easy and satisfying diagnosis to make. As with many patients suffering their first attack, there is relief that I will not be rolling up my shirt sleeves and reaching for the hacksaw but dismay that they should be burdened with (to paraphrase) "such an old fashioned malady of the affluent and the rich."

We all have uric acid coursing through our veins but relatively few of us suffer gout. When this acid occurs in excess it can form sharp crystals which settle within the joints. The inevitable result is exquisite tenderness, swelling and pain. Yuri Kassid had a build up of these uric acid crystals in the first joint of his big toe. This indeed is where three-quarters of all first attacks occur but they can arise within any joint, large or small. The crystals can also precipitate deep within the body, forming stones. These are unfortunately of a consistency that do not show on X-ray films and unlike kidney stones, for example, may remain undetected. Other gouty manifestations are soft tissue deposits on places such as the ear. These inflamed swellings are called tophi (as opposed to toffee-though rich food has a major role to play!)

Gout is both a genetic and dietary condition though some medicines, like diuretics, can bring it on. When I worked in New Zealand, Maori patients frequently referred to their condition as like having devils inside, munching away with razor-sharp fangs. Their Polynesian genetics coupled with the inviting but ruinous Western diet made gout a very common problem indeed. Rich foods such as red meat, chocolate, cheese and nuts should be kept to a minimum and alcoholic beverages including beer and wines, particularly port, are good at causing attacks.

The treatment of acute gout such as Yuri's is usually in the form of anti-inflammatories and Colchicine. This age-old medication is often effective but I always relay the adage to patients as I hand over the script that if Colchicine doesn't give you diarrhoea you are simply not taking it often enough. I've yet to have a patient who declined it in favour of continuing to suffer his pain. Once the attack has subsided the best Yuri can do is to drink plenty fluid, take more Vitamin C and avoid such rich foods as to which he had become accustomed. Should, despite this, he suffer several other incapacitating events I might suggest a long-term medicine called Allopurinol. This, by and large, lessens the frequency and severity of attacks. Its side-effects are minimal and rare and, again, few patients ever suggest dispensing with it, remembering the severity of their former symptoms.

Yuri, graciously accepted his prescription, donned his sock and limped from the room as uncomfortably as he entered, knowing he must make a few changes. First, he'd speak to his brother about the menu.

FAULTY WRITING

Scotland, as a nation, can boast about a few achievements and statistics but having the highest rate of Multiple Sclerosis in the world is surely not one of them. This is indeed, sadly, the case but for reasons that remain far from clear.

The actual condition, Multiple (or Disseminated) Sclerosis, was first identified centuries ago. It was observed that those with the condition tended to sustain inflammation and damage to the protective sheath that encases the brain and spinal cord (the Central Nervous System.) When this insulating material, similar to an electrical flex, becomes worn or frayed the messages sent and received by the brain become garbled or short-circuited. And so it was with my patient, Warren Cable. As is often the case, when MS first manifests in early adult life, Warren had a peculiar visual disturbance. He thought little of it at the time and indeed awoke a few mornings later to find it had rectified itself. A year or two later, he started to develop episodes of numbness and tingling in an arm or a leg. These never lasted terribly long and before his wife could convince him to seek a medical opinion the symptoms had invariably resolved or lessened. He often attributed these odd sensations to being cramped on public transport or lying awkwardly in bed. Eventually, he found himself stumbling and dropping objects and on one occasion scalded his hand with water from a recently boiled kettle. It had been entirely accidental but he said he watched it happen with "detached fascination and horror," for he had not felt a thing. By the time he did attend me in surgery, which almost required his wife using a cattle-prod to get him through the door (though he may not have felt even that!) I was more than a little suspicious. A Neurologist, the following week, was similarly concerned. Scans and a lumbar puncture demonstrated large patches of abnormality (or demyelination) where the nerve sheaths had partly disintegrated.

We do not know why this pathology should occur in some individuals and not in others. There may be an auto-immune element to the condition where the body essentially turns upon itself, causing damage for no apparent reason. It would seem that certain viruses are involved and, coupled with a probable genetic predisposition, problems arise. It is not simply a genetic or inheritable condition. A twin has a 30% lifetime chance of developing MS when his sibling already has been given the diagnosis.

More women than men have MS. It would be inaccurate to consider it as being one condition as there now several recognized subgroups. Warren's was the first type known as Relapsing Remitting and describes most people in the early stages of MS. Unpredictable attacks of weakness, numbness, spasms and balance problems occur. Recovery from each of these may be complete or partial. His reading into the subject had informed him that he may advance to the Secondary Progressive type and this was his fear. He was relieved his was not Primary Progressive, suffered by about 10%, this being the most aggressive type. This latter condition usually first occurs in older people and the physical decline is fairly steady, without episodes of remission or relief.

Warren and his wife Amy found the diagnosis difficult from the outset. After much thought, they decided to proceed that summer with a much anticipated holiday. Apart from anything else, the heat would do him good. They rightly informed the travel insurer of his new circumstances but found it was they who were rather "twitchy" about the situation. The insurance premium was effectively doubled. The copious forms that duly followed informed him that a surcharge would apply for wheelchairs and bags that may be required for continence care paraphernalia. Warren was almost symptom-free at that time but was rapidly discovering the difficulties he was about to face, well beyond any physical limitations.

Apart from the unpredictable nature of MS there are other uncertainties, from a medical point of view as well. Scans can be fairly diagnostic, but even identifying and locating patches of damage correlates poorly with the degree and type of disability present. Widespread demyelination may be seen in someone hardly aware of any problems and, conversely, severe disability may exist where very few irregularities are observed on the high-resolution scan images.

Warren and Amy knew there is no cure for the condition. High doses of steroids can lessen the severity of attacks but probably don't alter the long term course. Interferon treatment is for appropriate use in secondary progressive MS. This specific license may cause upset as patients and their families often feel they are being denied this expensive treatment for reasons of cost or rationing.

With good physical, psychological, medical and social support people with MS can live well and as long as anyone else. That is what I emphasized to Warren at that first meeting after his diagnosis and what I continue to help and encourage him to appreciate.

FACT OR FANTASY

Madge-Ann Narey had been sent along by her family to see me. She was, by her own admission, always a bit of a dreamer but they felt she increasingly dwelt in the past. For many, it can indeed be hard to distinguish fact from fantasy, romance from dispassion, truth from fable or actual from imagined.

The human mind has been compared to a computer but often its means of storage and retrieval are less objective. This is not necessarily a bad thing. Some people by their nature, perhaps mathematicians and accountants, deal better with numeric or factual data. Figures in, figures out. No more, no less. Others, of a more creative inclination; have images, memories and emotions conjured up by the merest, seemingly unrelated, incidents or items.

It is an utter delight to watch one's children or grandchildren play imaginatively. We might describe it as a cliché and waste of money when presents are discarded in favour of the packaging. I question the wisdom of parents who discourage belief in Santa Claus or never find time to read to their children.

As I drift into my twilight years, I find myself dwelling more on my formative years on this earth. I daresay my mind has embellished things a little and memories have been reshaped by viewing old photographic slides or by listening to family folklore. It is said that the sense of smell is the strongest trigger of memories. I recall with great fondness autumn afternoons helping Father stack the bonfire; filling the old Austin with 4-star or catching the waft from his briar pipe once the sun had set. Weekends included visits to dusty old churches and cathedrals, to the Polish shoemaker or to the coast by steam. I'm uncertain what these days of inhalation have done for my lungs but choose to ignore this in favour of the feelings of warmth and joy they give me still. I was described as an earnest little chatterbox who never exhausted telling tales of the farmyard, locomotives or superheroes. Pity, things have changed. Now, I can only relay to you tales from the surgery, rarely able to stray from the facts even if I so wished.

Some people's vivid imaginations may be used to bury painful memories. It seems, our rather fragile psyches cope best by attempting to erase traumatic thoughts or even replacing them with preferred, fictitious, ones. This is not confined to distant childhood events as some abused spouses display extraordinary denial of events, past or ongoing. Where criminal acts have occurred it is usually appropriate for the facts to be elucidated especially when others may continue to be subject to the same. I am not particularly in favour, as has been a modern trend, to unearth all hidden memories through hypnosis or psychoanalysis. When it is done for the purposes of entertainment there is utterly no excuse.

Advertisers and salespeople rely on (and exploit!) the public's imagination. "Put yourself in the position, sir, of winning this fabulous sum in the lottery." "Madam, envisage yourself luxuriating in this utterly gorgeous home. It is not just a house we offer you, oh no, but a lifestyle." We vote in the hope that the next politician will be better than the last. We give the benefit of considerable doubt, marvel at the manifesto pledges and allow our imagination to take over from logic and observed experience.

In our adversarial court system, lawyers may question a witness's interpretation of events, or more cynically seek to twist it. "At what speed did the accused's car smash into the unfortunate victim, my poor client over there?" The question was designed to create an image of recklessness and blame and ignored the fact my patient did all he could to avoid the drunk man who staggered onto the unlit road.

Some forms of illness make it hard to distinguish fact from fantasy. Schizophrenia, head injury, autism and dementia may each manifest in an inability to see things for what they are or to seriously misinterpret the world in which we live.

Various intoxicants, particularly drugs and alcohol, may either contribute to the above or themselves blur the boundaries of reality. The medicines we prescribe are often not free from side-effects; including delirium, confusion and hallucination.

Some of our greatest works of art and literature are said to have been created under the influence of intoxicants or mental illness. Van Gogh, Hemmingway and Woolf were all geniuses with tortured souls, and ultimately took their own lives. Although he only bordered on the eccentric, Albert Einstein once said that "Imagination is more important than knowledge."

Religious belief and experience in themselves are dismissed by some as lacking in evidence or not being up to the rigours of scientific scrutiny. For believers, this is their step of faith and of little consequence to their views. They may even welcome historical or archaeological evidence as it emerges to substantiate, at least in part, centuries old scripture. Few, I think, regard ancient religious text as 100% accurate and rather enjoy the poetic and paraphrased interpretations of widely accepted events and characters.

I was not convinced Madge-Ann had a problem at all. In all the years I've known her, I have enjoyed her musings and writings. She says she is living her dream and can return to reality whenever she wishes, but prefers the meanderings of her own mind.

I just wish my subconsciousness was half as fertile and exciting.

TIME BOMBS

Eck Splode had been visiting his wife in hospital when he collapsed. He remembered little of the incident but did recall that he developed very severe lower back pain shortly before things went black. Here he was, sitting in surgery some three weeks later, wanting to know the details. Eck had suffered a ruptured abdominal aortic aneurysm (AAA.)

The aorta is the main blood vessel of the body. It it the artery which comes out the top of the heart, loops round and down, passes through the diaphragm and divides in two before reaching the pelvis and legs.

As is the case in some 6% of all men over sixty-five, he had developed a ballooning in the lower part of the blood vessel. This had been unknown to him, and me, and is sadly usually the case in such aneurysms, when they first make themselves apparent by rupturing. The aorta has the thickness and pressure similar to that of a garden hose. As can be imagined, the leakage of blood is often catastrophic. Four out of five people who suffer a sudden tear do not make it to discuss the details afterwards with their doctors or anyone else, save perhaps, St Peter.

Visitors to hospitals have the rather annoying tendency of taking unwell themselves. The combination of emotion and heat seems to lead to an alarming number of faints and funny turns. An alert staff nurse on the ward quickly realized Mr Splode's collapse was more serious and he was transferred to theatre within minutes. The surgeon made a rapid incision, immersed his hands in Eck's blood-filled abdomen and soon located the source of the pulsating, heavy bleed. After dozens of units of blood were transfused, the aorta was clamped, the flow stemmed and a synthetic graft replaced the offending split blood vessel. He spent a few days in intensive care, then he and Mary (who was only in for a minor surgical procedure) returned home together on the same day.

"The surgeon said these aneurysms are like timebombs. How long would I have had it, Dr Ken?" It was a good question Eck asked. Most aneurysms cause no symptoms whatsoever, even when quite large. They tend to expand by about 10% each year and, as might be predicted, the larger they are the more likely rupture is to occur. They are most often discovered incidentally: when we are examining the abdomen for other reasons or X-raying the bowel, for instance. "But should all us older chaps not be scanned to detect these aneurysms?" I fully agree that there should indeed be a screening programme in place certainly for men, where AAAs are a good deal more common. Aneurysm rupture is the 13th most common cause of death (unlucky for all!) in this country. Planned (elective) repairs, though not without their own serious risks, could save many lives. If a smaller aneurysm is discovered it does not necessarily mean repair should take place. The likelihood of a small one bursting is minimal but monitoring over succeeding years would be crucial. Actual elective repair these days is less complex than it used to be. Previously, as in the emergency situation, a section of aorta was removed and replaced with a synthetic graft. Now, a stent is passed up through the groin and is placed as an inner sleeve, within the swollen aneurysm. This is a much simpler, safer technique which is improving all the time.

Eck Splode survived his exploding time bomb. He is just grateful it occurred in the best place possible. Thanks to the quick actions of the nursing and medical staff the "detonation" did not lead to his expiration or indeed his cremation. Instead, he now has more time than nature might have intended.

UP PERISCOPE

It's almost that time again. I can't say I look forward to it, but know that it has to be done. The time when doctor becomes patient; dignity becomes immaterial and all becomes clear.

Once every two years, this particular chap receives through the post a sachet that can only be described as "dynamite for the bowels." After the supreme cleansing process occurs, he takes the day off work and motors to the Infirmary. Once there, he is asked politely to drop his drawers for the purposes of having his colon/bowel examined. The procedure of colonoscopy is, to inner space, what astronomy is to the outer variety. One is examined from bottom (literally!) to top, from outside to inside and from left to right. Fortunately, the lengthy, flexible scope used is increasingly sophisticated and of a narrower gauge than it was previously. The fibre-optic tube has a viewing piece at the operator's end and at the other there is the clever ability to negotiate the corners, contours and folds of one's tortuous gut. The experience is not limited to the specialist carrying out the procedure. All present can now share, in an educational fashion, this "inner adventure" by watching proceedings live on a monitor. Call it morbid fascination if you like, but I am amongst those intrigued enough to observe as every wrinkle and polyp is scrutinised and sampled, as necessary. I do pay my licence fee after all.

I could no more choose my genes than anyone else and just happen to be a member of a family that has an increased incidence of colonic cancer. After seeing relatives succumb in their middle years to this dreadful condition and, myself having reached a certain age, measures have to be taken. By "measures," I mean approximately 4 or 5 feet of large bowel is carefully examined, inch by inch.

There are more deaths from cancer of the bowel in this country than from any other origin, except that of the lung. It is for this reason that bashfulness or a certain distaste about talking about one's bowel habit ought to be overcome. I find patients are either rather too keen to talk about their bowels or are a bit too reluctant. In those with a veritable enthusiasm, they likely have had recent or repeated examinations and when there is the slightest degree of constipation or looseness, their imaginations run riot. But I fear more for the latter, less complaining, type of patient who may start by saying "it is probably nothing and is rather an embarrassing problem doctor, but..." I often objectively state that it certainly isn't embarrassing for me (without divulging the need for my own biannual examinations) as I discuss such things each day. I have seen and heard it all, as it were, and if my face is red it is only from weathering and age.

Bowel cancer is readily treatable, if discovered early enough. Such screening and surveillance programmes as mine, mean that when/if cancerous growths are discovered the offending portion of colon can be chopped out. Chemotherapy or radiotherapy may follow, determined by the stage of the disease and on what the oncologist advises. Depending on the actual location, adjacent ends of cut bowel may be sutured together or one end brought to the surface in the form of a stoma/colostomy. The degree of cancer of the bowel (erosion of the bowel wall) is graded by the Dukes system. This bears no relation to the fine gentlemen of Buccleuch, Hamilton or Roxburghe but to one Cuthbert Duke and his classification of colorectal tumours in 1932.

Colonoscopy is not just used to detect bowel cancer. Various other pathologies can be diagnosed or assessed. Inflammatory conditions such as Crohn's disease or Ulcerative Colitis need ongoing monitoring as well, when of a more serious nature.

For some conditions, especially where it is difficult to determine the source of bleeding, technology is advancing. A small camera-capsule is swallowed and it takes a series of pictures during transit. It is hoped the miniature spy-camera is retrieved from the pan, as technicians have no particular desire to study our sewerage systems, even from the comfort and sterility of the laboratory.

I hope to be given the all-clear for another 24 months but know to re-attend sooner if symptoms warrant. I am not quite on first name terms with the ancillary staff in the department but Dr Perry Schcoppe, my gastroenterologist, has become a familiar face. I daresay, it is not my face he has committed to memory!

THE CHOCHOLIC

Most people enjoy a slice of chocolate. Some enjoy it more than others, and some much more than others. Candy Barr fell (or would have happily dived into a vat) in the latter category. Her consumption, however, exceeded what would ever be considered reasonable and so recently, as with every other month, she attended to discuss and describe her desire for chocolate.

On her first consultation, I sat back almost hypnotized. I listened to her graphically and quite deliciously describe her wont, her want and her "need" to consume the luxurious brown stuff, in abundance. Soon, rather than her visits being akin to commercial breaks amidst the more serious and mundane aspects of my day, her habit struck me more as an addiction and a cause for concern. She was not a particularly happy person but nor was she depressed.

Each evening after returning from work, she would ensure the children's homework was done, then prepare a "healthy" evening meal. Once the wee ones were tucked up in bed, the "cravings" would commence. She would say to Mr Barr that she needed some air but took the opportunity to nip down to the local convenience store. Soon afterwards, she returned with a carrier bag laden with "goodies and treats." She would find a further excuse and steal upstairs. Once there, the wrappers and packaging were torn off and the feasting began. So it was, each and every evening. There were some chocolate bars and sweets she preferred to others, but all were better than none. The first few megapacks and the two-for-one slabs seemed to satisfy the initial craving, but she didn't stop there.

Candy said she hated herself for; the secrecy and the shame, the expense and the effect. She did not nibble for nourishment, but gorged out of greed for the stuff. Any initial positive effects were quickly negated by the enormous sugar and fat load to which she daily subjected herself. Her weight was systematically increasing, her skin getting greasier and her self-esteem was plummeting.

I tried to reason with her by suggesting she ration herself. In the Moody family, "Sunday chocolate" is a throwback to the post-war years when rationing was a reality. Nowadays, it is ubiquitous and entire shops are dedicated to the worship of this confectionery. It has become a central part of almost every festival, including Mothers' Day, Valentine's Day, Easter and Christmas.

Candy recognized that she had a problem. The trouble was that I was not convinced how keen she was to properly address it. I felt her so-called addiction could be overcome with a bit of self-control and, by definition, only she could exercise this.

In moderation, chocolate is considered to convey certain health benefits. It may lower blood pressure and LDL cholesterol and dark chocolate often contains anti-oxidants. It can increase serotonin levels in the brain-which may increase mood and the feeling of wellbeing. Perhaps this surge, like the hit alcoholics and drug addicts get from their fix, is what makes people return time and again, despite the often devastating consequences. I tried warning Candy that she may induce diabetes and other problems of being overweight. I played the emotional card by reminding her that child labour and other exploitation occurs in the Ivory Coast where the bulk of the world's cocoa is harvested. I was not getting through.

On her last visit, she described problems and losses that had occurred among her family and friends. She detailed how she had given greatly of her time and resources to see these loved ones through bereavement, serious illness and separation. This had put issues in perspective, she said, and helped her see how damaging her behaviour had become. She had gone the extra mile (but this time, not for chocolate!)

I assured her I had never considered her a fruit, a nut or a flake but pointed out I had contributed little to the situation. She still has dark days, just not of the chocolate variety. Candy Barr looked and felt better. She had benefited from an emotional boost of sorts rather than a sugar one.

AN UNKNOWN PATIENT

On a cold Monday morning, the local ambulance crew called the surgery to say it was attending a sudden death. Mondays, statistically, are the commonest time of the week to die but, being only a moderate sized practice, we are not summoned to many unexpected demises. It is also the busiest time of the week in surgery but I knew I should make my way to the house as soon as practicable. The paramedics would be awaiting my arrival but, more importantly, there were likely shocked relatives to see as well. I apologized to the packed waiting room and donned my coat again.

Not recognizing the deceased's name or even the particular address, I wondered if this lady might have been visiting from another area. I asked a receptionist to retrieve the medical notes but her hasty search proved fruitless. I motored across town and parked behind the ambulance. One green-clad paramedic was in the sitting room with the newly widowed husband and the other accompanied me to the room above. My "patient" was indeed dead, probably only for a couple of hours. She was peaceful and seemed to have slipped away in her sleep. I made a general examination of the body, declared life extinct and took a note of the time. Legally, it is only doctors who can declare patients dead, except in cases of decapitation or decomposition – though neither malefaction or putrefaction was suspected.

It emerged that Ann O'Nymas's husband had gone to take his wife a cup of tea, as was their custom, but found her unresponsive and cold. He dropped the cup and in a panic rang the three digits, rarely used but known to all. The ambulance was quickly at his door but it was apparent that Ann was beyond resuscitation and attempts would have been futile.

Over a cup of tea (freshly brewed), Mr O'Nymas recounted how he had been concerned for his wife's health over the weekend. Her cough had been increasingly chesty and she spent much of Sunday sleeping in front of the telly. It wasn't like her, he said, as she never normally missed the programme about antiques. He had offered to call a doctor but she forbade. She hadn't even bothered with her wretched cigarettes. Noting the photographs of grandchildren in local school uniforms, I asked how long they had lived in the house. I was astonished to hear it had been almost forty years. How had they never been known to me? A few townsfolk travel elsewhere for their medical care but I assumed I knew everyone in the practice and have probably been in every home, over the years. Not so, seemingly. It wasn't that they were a private couple, indeed Ann had a passion for needlecraft and dance, and certificates and awards were evidence enough of her skill.

It emerged, that years ago a doctor had failed to recognize her sister's diphtheria and the consequences were profound. Ann had developed a dislike and suspicious attitude to any form of medical care and sought her own remedies and tonics, when required. She had never darkened our door or even crossed our path, astonishingly, during her confinements with the children. They were now grown up and the one living locally was a vaguely familiar name.

Some patients consult us every week in life; this seems to be whether they need to or not. Such doctor dependence or illness behaviour is, ironically, not very healthy and, I have noticed, tends to transfer to their offspring.

It would certainly be a rather paternalistic relationship I would have with this town if I really were to know, and be familiar with, every single person. In truth, I thought I did! It is almost refreshing to discover that some people can grow up, raise families, work, socialize, live and dare I say die yet remain unknown to me. Society is indeed made up of people and not just patients.

I could not simply issue a death certificate for Ann. She had essentially been anonymous to me and I could not confidently state a cause of death. To this end, as it were, I called the duty police surgeon and procurator fiscal to discuss the case. It seemed to me, however, she had died of pneumonia. Her lifelong smoking habit would have contributed but her aversion and avoidance of doctors may literally have been the death of her. Had she been seen earlier, the sounding of her chest would likely have determined the seriousness of her condition and treatment, perhaps hospital admission, might have made a difference. We'll never know.

RAT POISON

"How're ye farin' on yon Warfarin?" So goes my usual question, in the vernacular, to those newly on this particular prescribed drug. My clumsy play on words is probably wearing as thin as one's blood, when on an anticoagulant medicine.

Rod Dent was one such patient who found himself, after cardiac surgery, taking the wee pills on a daily basis. He was indeed correct in observing that Warfarin is what farmers and others have used for decades to kill the vermin *Rattus Norvegicus* and its darker cousin *Rattus Rattus*. Warfarin interferes with Vitamin K in the blood and makes it less likely and less able to clot. When sufficient quantities are consumed, the beasties haemorrhage internally and literally bleed to death.

Now that Rod was on this "poison", he was keen not to be a pest (and we never saw him as such!) but knew he would need to attend the surgery on a regular basis from now on. The necessary blood tests, or INRs, measure the degree of thinning of the blood and the dose of the medicine is adjusted accordingly. He also knew he was no lab rat or guinea pig and ever increasing numbers of our patients are on this particular treatment- though I wouldn't go so far as to say we are plagued!

Many elderly (and some not so elderly) people are recognized as having the condition atrial fibrillation (AF.) This is where the heart instead of beating in a regular rhythm, twitches, rather like the thrashing tail of a certain rodent when enraged. The rate of a fibrillating heart can be reduced by another of nature's potential poisons, Digitalis; though this is less important. The danger of such random beats is that blood, rather than entering and leaving the heart every second or so, is allowed to pool and form eddies. When this occurs it is much more likely to form clots. These either clog the heart itself or may be projected from the cardiac chambers, out and along the ever-narrowing arterial system, where they eventually lodge and block. The brain and lungs are the most commonly affected organs and the damage can be catastrophic. Sometimes, doctors are only alerted to the problems of atrial fibrillation and clot formation after stroke or pulmonary embolism has occurred. The hope of Warfarin treatment then would be to break up the clot in the short term and minimize the chances of recurrence in the future. AF and artificial heart valve replacement are the main reasons for being on Warfarin for the rest of one's days. A deep venous thrombosis (DVT) of the leg usually only requires six months of treatment, unless it were to become a recurring problem.

I've always felt, Warfarin and its regular monitoring is rather less than sophisticated. Even in the most stable of conditions, people need to have INR blood tests at least every six weeks. Not only is this costly and time consuming but, due to the unpredictable nature of Warfarin, people may be over or under anti-coagulated between tests. It would be preferable to have a much more stable and controlled blood-thinning agent and I know research is taking place into this very subject.

Numerous medicines, supplements and tonics can interfere with Warfarin, either enhancing or antagonizing its effect. Anti-inflammatory drugs, even Aspirin, should be avoided as the combination of an ulcer-promoter and a blood-thinner could quickly leave you stiff and having four little limbs pointing upwards. Alcohol, does not necessarily need to be avoided but intake should be at a rather steady (and modest) level. Consumption should never be heavy as this would greatly affect Warfarin's action. Furthermore, falls and injuries to the head and elsewhere could cause serious internal bleeding. There are some people, in whom the risk of falling is just so great or their lifestyles so chaotic that it is may be relatively safer for them not to be on Warfarin at all.

"Will I be able to live a full life, now I'm on this wretched rat poison?" asked Rod, a little anxiously. I believe he already has led a fuller life than most but reassured him that with close monitoring and common sense he will likely live well beyond the lifespan of the average rat, some 21 months. He knows the "poison" has to be temporarily stopped prior to dental or other surgery and views the situation with due respect.

"One last question, Dr Ken; if I'm more likely to bleed, will I still be able to shave?"

I looked at Rod Dent and commented to the effect that he certainly could, with care, but his were indeed the finest whiskers I've seen in a long time.

SOLDIERS AS PATIENTS

Rankin Fyle had served his time in the army and now sat in surgery discussing what his next venture in life might be. I say he sat, but in fact only did so when instructed and preceded each reply to my questions with "Sir." I could see that life in civvy street was not necessarily going to be straightforward for this former squaddie.

I've never worn a soldier's hat or beret in any official capacity but I take my head covering off to those who have served in the Forces. Some of my patients are former navy and air force personnel but I seem to meet far more chaps who served their time in the army. When I first started in general practice, we had many veterans of the Great War but they are all marching on the great parade ground in the sky. Even survivors of the Second War are now, at least, octogenarians and becoming ever fewer on the ground.

One does not need to be old, of course, to have retired from active service. Injury, illness and, occasionally, inglorious dismissal may cause military personnel to become patients, asking to enrol on a list of a rather different kind.

I have noticed that many ex-servicemen choose to work in the charitable sector. My reading of this is that they are efficient, hard-working and prepared to live in climates and areas of the world less appealing to others. Sometimes, they tell me, they are fulfilling a promise made to themselves to contribute to the welfare and security of people, but in a somewhat different and perhaps more humanitarian capacity.

I have respect for soldiers in other ways too. This is not a saluting, heel-clicking sort of respect but a quiet admiration. It is refreshing to hear their directness in speech and thought. A soldier tends to say what he means and means what he says (if you know what I mean!) As doctors, we are aware that some patients have difficulty expressing themselves or articulating problems, whether of a personal nature or not. A series of more minor issues may indicate a deeper, unspoken problem and there may be a deal of unravelling for us to do. Never so with soldiers. To them, a spade is a spade; a symptom is a symptom and a problem needs sorted. The sooner the better and he'll do anything he can to assist.

A soldier's more choice use of terms in the vernacular may not be appreciated by more delicate ears but is rarely offensive. It has been said a soldier swears an oath of allegiance to God and the queen and doesn't stopping swearing thereafter; like the proverbial trooper, I suppose. I don't know if this is true but, when under attack, it will be ammunition a soldier reaches for rather than adjectives; guns rather than grammar and protection rather than punctuation.

Many ex-servicemen do seem to pack up their troubles in ageing kit-bags but not all can do so with such ease. Mental ill-health, the effects of stress and even suicide are problems for which doctors should be vigilant. It is always a great disappointment to soldiers when they meet apparent indifference and squandered life back here at home. They express bewilderment when people forget what real freedom means and that it is literally worth fighting for. Soldiers are involved in situations and witness sights that most of us are spared but, as fit and well-trained as they might be, under the fatigues they are flesh and blood too.

Much military deployment at present around the world is in a peace-keeping or preventative role. Politics is always the driving force behind modern conflicts but the motives are often called into question. Support for causes overseas vary as armchair observers postulate that battles are fought on false premises and with undeclared objectives, often for the acquisition of natural resources. I too find it difficult to understand why armies mobilize against certain tyrants and threats, yet turn blind eyes to atrocities elsewhere in the world, most often in Africa. What should not waver though is our support for the thousands of troops serving abroad. All decent people have considerable sympathy for the families when we see flag-draped coffins being carried slowly by comrades up church steps. I write this as I look at the front page photograph of a young local man, killed in action in Afghanistan.

I learned recently that 1968 was the only year in the twentieth century that a British serviceman was not lost in action. We remember the fallen, each November, at the commemoration of Armistice Day but should be ever mindful and grateful.

Rankin is only too aware how much he and his comrades gave, and took, from their experiences. He knows he is fortunate and that it is time now for him to move on. He had always dreamt of opening a florist's shop on the High St and has just put down a deposit.

WHERE THE GRASS IS GREENER

I am always interested to hear why people decide to emigrate. As often as once each month, I chat with patients about their plans for permanent departure. And so it was with Colin Neil and his wife Peri Neil (she promised to always stick by him.) Colin and Peri felt that they had a run of bad luck in recent years. Their business had failed and, without beating about the bush, they "cared too much to witness the destructive path down which our nation's leaders are taking us." His great-uncle had adopted the colonial way of life almost a century before, for reasons he compared to his own. Colin's family was young enough, they felt, to adapt to the changes that lay ahead.

I don't usually have much of a role to play in emigration proceedings. The laborious form-filling and hoop jumping are left to the applicants themselves and I suppose the bureaucracy is a means of testing the strength of one's resolve. I had been asked to perform a fairly thorough medical and confirmed that Colin and his family are not likely to be exporting more than just their skills. Chest X-Rays are almost standard and are a ready way of determining whether active TB is present. They would also indicate if an undiagnosed tumour is about to rear its ugly head and I suspect, from a purely financial perspective, most governments would decline an applicant who was going to require costly medical care as soon as he reached their shores.

I think I've only once been asked my views about an "uprooting" but of course would be loathe to venture an opinion as to whether a venture across the globe is in one's best interests. Even if I knew a person well I would hesitate to opine on, perhaps, the biggest decision he might ever make. We tend not to hear about the more successful emigrations but every so often are reacquainted with former patients. The promised or anticipated lifestyle may not always be realised and, even when it is, people can find the strangeness of fresh pastures, the language barrier and the separation from families back home comes at too high a price.

It would seem wise not to sell lock, stock and barrel in the event that the adopted country's fields are less fertile and leas less luscious than had been imagined. After all, it is only chlorophyll that makes grass greener. A recognizance trip would seem advisable but this may not be financially practicable and a greater leap of faith is required.

In the old days, people were driven from the land, as in the Highland Clearances. They were turfed out their rented properties and left homeless and hopeless. At other times, when economic or agricultural disaster struck, people left Scotland for the last time. Even for the more affluent, word of opportunities in the New World was too much to resist and the relative comfort here was abandoned for the expectation of greater prosperity abroad. Crossing the Atlantic or other oceans was an eventful and risky business. Shipwreck and disease meant, for many, that the anticipated new life was not life at all.

Scots are greatly respected throughout the world. Our inventive, industrious, philanthropic and literate forefathers enabled progress in many fields and the names of Telford, Bell, Fleming, McAdam, Smith, Carnegie, Scott and Burns still carry much influence. I also think being seen as the "underdog" to our much larger southerly neighbour has something to do with it too!

One aspect of emigration that amuses as much as it amazes me is the strength of the Scottish expat community. People seem to hold onto their dearest memories, perhaps neglecting the less pleasant ones or even forgetting the reasons for their departure in the first place. Rather than diminish, the strength of feeling can intensify in second and third generation emigrants (perhaps they have never experienced our cold, dreich weather!) Scots have always been able to recount stories with great affection and romanticism and our history is nothing if not involved.

Nowadays, communication and transportation are so much more efficient and our world indeed seems to shrink. Visiting relations at the other side of the planet is a cheaper form of holiday when accommodation is provided. Cheap telephone calls and free web chats mean that people are often in touch more than when they lived within yards of each other. Emigration is not truly the one-way ticket it once was.

I reread Colin and Peri's postcard from New Zealand and wondered upon the odds of their return. Good luck to them. I hope they find the peace and prosperity they deserve.

ECCENTRICS

Weir Dow was nothing if not an interesting fellow. His preference was for a long burgundy velvet coat, army camouflage trousers and a leopard skin fez atop his balding head. He was tall with shoulder-length hair, a crooked nose and had the longest finger nails I've probably ever seen. His spectacles were held together with masking tape and one lens was badly cracked. They usually hung from his neck by a boot lace. This frayed cord had not been replaced on his left boot but that hardly mattered as his footwear rarely matched. Other from that, Weir would not have stood out in a crowd! This hypothesis, however, would probably not be put to the test as he shunned gatherings of all sorts and people in general.

I did not often cross paths with Weir or venture up his overgrown driveway. His large house had seen and enjoyed better days and maintenance was clearly not high on his list of priorities. Indeed, for a while he had been the victim of taunting from local boys and most of the panes in the greenhouses were smashed. He had lived alone in his sprawling Victorian villa since his mother's death and I doubt there would have been many visitors, save the occasional delivery man seeking directions.

Weir had never worked in any official capacity but seemingly had a brilliant mind. All had gone well in his early years; he excelled at school and received a bursary to study Mathematics and Physics at university. Sadly, he didn't manage to cope with the attendant pressures. It was said that alcohol, drugs and weeks of sleepless nights wrestling with formulae and equations had simply fried his brain.

The answers on his end of year exam papers were described by the professors as "utter gibberish" and poor Weir was duly thrown out of the establishment. Nowadays, efforts would be made to explore the reasons behind such a downward spiral but forty years ago mental illness was even less well understood than it is today. His parents had taken him to a psychiatrist and schizophrenia was eventually diagnosed. Weir dismissed the prescribed medication, describing it as "intolerable and unnecessary." When he learned that his psychiatrist had retired, he refused to see anyone else, quite literally. His medical records show that my predecessors made attempts to visit him over the following year or two but were met with hostility, resentment and, occasionally, violence. He was never felt, though, to be of sufficient risk to be detained against his will. The townspeople were not particularly sympathetic to the plight of the family but kirk elders and a few others called out of kindness, or perhaps curiosity. The rare sightings of the Dows around the area became ever rarer.

Eccentrics, as we tend to label people such as Weir, are those who depart from normal accepted forms of behaviour. They are often considered bizarre or odd individuals. Rather literally, they may inhabit the margins of society though not necessarily as recluses. Sometimes, society appreciates and finds it refreshing that such "characters" exist. Those who fly in the face of convention and so-called normality may be applauded for their originality and individualism; especially when creativity or artistic brilliance is the result.

Perceived eccentricity may result from one's upbringing. If parents are flighty, capricious, unpredictable, obsessive, pernickety or mercurial it is quite possible that such traits are learned or seen as accepted patterns of behaviour. It is my belief that many eccentrics, as in Weir's case, suffer from forms of mental illness. Schizophrenia most often presents in one's late teens or early twenties and this indeed is when one is subject to considerable change. Such pressures may precipitate a condition that was bubbling under the surface.

Early recognition and treatment and ongoing support are essential for successful return to proper functioning and the realizing of potential, in whatever form that may take. Many people, who suffer schizophrenia at its full delusional intensity, are observed in later life to be "burnt out" and subject to more negative features, including withdrawal and depression. This may be a combination of both the effects of medication and a natural progession of the illness.

Autism and Asperger's syndrome are conditions more often associated with childhood, when schooling is disrupted or frankly impossible. Such children, of course, don't simply overcome their problems on reaching adulthood and often slide down the social and economic ladder.

I was able to give such a vivid description of Weir's appearance because I had the pleasure of having tea with him recently. I can't pretend I didn't consider the cleanliness of the cup, as I watched him blow the dust off his late mother's finest tea-set. Out of the blue, the surgery had received a call from him asking me to visit. He had politely declined to give a reason. Normally, we would need further information before downing tools but, as normality is not a term easily attributed to Weir, I was happy to make an exception. It emerged that he felt he was dying. He had summoned his solicitor for later that afternoon and wished to settle his affairs. He did not particularly need my confirmation of his predicted impending demise but felt it may be beneficial for legal purposes. I convinced him an examination and blood tests would assist in my assessment. He gestured his assent by waving a dirty lace handkerchief and promptly coughed into it.

Two days later, I returned and confirmed my initial suspicion that Weir had pneumonia and antibiotics should see him right. I have my doubts he took what I prescribed but I continue to visit him, now, on an annual basis. Each time I take with me my own milk.

PART 5

PRACTICE MATTERS

ALL-WEATHER DOCTOR

"I missed my last appointment, Dr Ken. The rain was terrible that day." I wasn't sure if April Schauerz was simply declaring these two statements as fact or offering some form of cryptic apology. I am no longer irritated, rather amused, when the merest hint of precipitation seems to have miraculous healing properties or suddenly nullifies the need for medical attention. Of course, if old Mrs Forsten-Gale is likely to be blown down the street like tumbleweed and is genuinely in need, I'll make every effort to visit.

Despite what we might claim, I think we rather enjoy the unpredictability of the elements. Comments such as: "Foul weather we're having" or "Getting colder" are often ice-breakers to conversation or used as simple pleasantries. In terms of deeper substance and sincerity though, they are almost as light as nimbostratus cloud formations. One rather introverted patient Mr Rockall Malin, given half a chance, would relay to me the unabridged shipping forecast for the next twenty-four hours. As much as I enjoy the melodic, almost poetic, recital on the wireless, preceding the news, it is not my idea of fun at a dinner party.

I've known expatriates to move back to Scotland having found the predictably high temperatures in the Colonies "unbearably monotonous." They discovered the greener grass to be scorched, or perhaps it was just a mirage all along. I confess to being an impromptu amateur forecaster when out strolling. As a local GP and well-kent (and weathered) face, an innocent "How are you?" may be taken as more than a rhetorical question and I am still standing, listening to the Storr-McLeods detailing their every ailment, twenty minutes later. It may not be just the dogs straining at the leash to get away. If I left my Sou'wester hanging next to the barometer in the porch, because the needle was stuck at "Fair", I will indeed have a fair excuse to leave Mrs Raine Storr-McLeod to dry up mid sentence and consult me, more appropriately, on Monday morning. She might feel a little under the weather but so might I, literally.

During winter months I have found myself helping local farmers dig sheep out from snow drifts before trudging my way to surgery in galloshes or hitching a lift on a tractor.

Surgeries in the summer months are often quieter. There are several reasons for this, including patients being away on vacation. Visitors to the town, other than elderly ladies tumbling out of coaches or forgetting their medication, rarely seem to need our medical assistance . People generally feel better and feel better about themselves when the sun is shining. Seasonal Affective Disorder (SAD) is of course rather appropriately named and studies consistently show consultation rates for depression are greater in winter months then in summer ones.

Someone once said that there is no such thing as bad weather, just the wrong type of clothing. Assuming this was not a simple advertising slogan for protective outdoor gear, therein lies some wisdom. Cancelled beach or golf trips due to inclement conditions are undoubtedly disappointing, ruined harvests can be catastrophic but in some ways weather is just weather. I mentioned summer and winter months but am increasingly convinced by the notion that the climate is changing, driven by our seemingly insatiable need for fossil fuels. I would postulate that the words "unseasonal" and "unseasonable" will disappear from dictionaries as the seasons become less distinct and we come to accept and expect aberrant conditions. ("Unseasoned" is likely to remain in use as I suspect condiments will always be necessary for more discerning palates!)

So, Miss Schauerz, a bit of drizzle kept you away did it? Far be it from me to criticise your fair-weather affectations, but come rain or shine; hail or high water; pestilence, famine or flood I'll be here as usual, healing the sick and listening to tales of woe (during extended office hours anyway!)

STRIPPED OF A JOB

"You know of course that each evening, once she pulls down the shutters of the surgery, she goes and pulls down other things." I did not, at first, follow. A slightly grubby patient, Mr Kleip, had information to which he felt we should be party. "Your Beryl Esk's a pole dancer!" I soon gathered he was not suggesting Beryl's skills lay in merry English folk dancing in early May or polkas customary to Poland. Had I not been so pole-axed by this revelation, I might have asked how he had specifically acquired such a fact and whether Mrs Kleip would have approved.

It emerged that Beryl, our friendly and reliable receptionist, felt it necessary to supplement her income by peeling off garments in nightclubs in the city. The practice manager, my colleagues and I discussed this rather delicate matter and arranged a private meeting with Beryl (in the surgery, you understand!) To a certain extent, what she did with her time was her own business but the concern remained that the name of the practice may have been brought into disrepute.

Beryl was not particularly surprised to be called to the meeting. She said she knew it was only a matter of time before her cover was blown and the goggle-eyed Mr Kleip in the front row was unmistakable. We were not going to tear a strip off her and, on this occasion, it was her soul that she bared. She was a single mum, having been deserted by her husband, and had to consider the children's future. I had some sympathy and knew the remuneration at the surgery was modest but was surprised she had to resort to such...immodesty. She was not exactly skint but showing skin was how she apparently managed to make ends meet. This, she argued, kept the wolves (but not their whistles!) from the door.

We had always found Beryl good at the front desk but being so up front was rather too much. It would only be a matter of time before the cheaper end of the press would pay scant regard to reputations and headlines like "Swapping hassles for tassels" or "Next please, Sexed please" were not the sort of exposure the practice, or indeed Beryl, needed. She was insistent that what she did was not prostitution but accepted it wasn't entirely innocent either.

Even if the practice budget allowed, we couldn't have offered her a pay rise sufficient to dissuade her from disrobing. This, on principle, would send the wrong message. It is unlikely our other, older, receptionists would necessarily step on the stage to the same type of applause but we had to consider public decency!

As doctors we take ultimate responsibility for the actions and behaviour of our employees in work and, to an extent, out of work as well. We could not condone Beryl's rather dubious second occupation but made it clear that she was welcome to remain at the practice, on the condition that any alternative sources of income involved a greater deal of attire. It was either our patients or her punters, but not both. She appreciated our offer but sadly declined. She left us no alternative, she would have to go-go.

FUNERAL DIRECTORS

"I am always grateful when I receive a calendar. Some years, I may be given more than one. They tend to be from pharmaceutical companies or local businesses. Ideally, it would arrive a few months before the new year so that future appointments and meetings may be penned in, as appropriate. I never quite understood why one particular glossy flip book takes until February each year before delivery to the surgery. I suppose you could say, like everything else about Mr Graves a local undertaker, being late is his business. (This would be a catchy but rather irreverent slogan, but better than "At your disposal," I'd contend!) In fact, each page simply states "Doug Graves. Funeral Director."

I'm not sure why Doug feels the need to advertise. Business always has a way of finding its way to his door. Long ago, I came to a conclusion (not literally obviously!) that there was something a little unseemly about a doctor displaying a calendar, or anything else for that matter, advertising a funeral director. If a patient were to ask me what long-term prognosis I might give him, and during my deliberations his eyes fell on such a calendar, he may suspect the worst. Undertakers' calendars may also imply a degree of clairvoyance. One practice secretary was tempted to flick nervously through the pages, expecting to see the saints' days and bank holidays replaced with anticipated certain "expiry dates."

You might also wonder what twelve images a funeral director would choose. Headstones, during different seasons and in different lights, may be of interest to one selecting a piece of granite from a specialist catalogue but would not give me any particular inspiration at the start of each working day. Mourners would not be suitable subject matter either and would be entitled to direct stern looks at Doug were he to point a camera in their direction at any stage in the proceedings. His images, instead, are usually of rural Scottish scenes; sheep running across frosty fields or castles perched next to lochs.

It is rather important for a GP practice, in these smaller communities, to get along well with local undertakers. This is not just because Doug is likely to do me the honours should my trumpet call be heard before his, but because our work overlaps to an extent. We speak or meet professionally every week or two and our dealings with bereaved families should be as professional, informed and courteous as possible. Doug and his assistants, Paul Behrer and M. Balmer, were originally carpenters who could turn their hand to anything. They discovered that making coffins was more lucrative. Doug's brother, N Graves, is a monumental sculptor. He is reputedly able to knock off an epitaph faster than anyone else in the trade but his spelling and grammar are a little less impressive. His response when criticized is that, for centuries, his predecessors wrote "f" rather than "s" or chiselled their speech impediments such as, "Here lyeth." It apparently took him two years to realize that this town was not the capital offence centre of the country just because almost every ancient tombstone states that the departed had "asked his executors" to inter him where he now lies.

The business of death is changing. A local undertaker finds it somewhat of an undertaking, as it were, being on-call round the clock. For this reason people who die when the parlour is closed may have their bodies uplifted by a larger funeral organization, most likely based in the city. This is leading to a less personal service, I daresay, but I do have sympathy (not just for the bereaved) but for Doug & Co. as GPs also found ourselves unable to cater for all, at all times and still be at our best.

Funerals are generally less formal and sombre and are treated more as celebrations of life. Often now, in accordance with the deceased's wishes, "mourners" are instructed to wear bright colours and to laugh rather than cry. Good undertakers will try to accommodate requests and deal with all matters large and small, with dignity and respect. One company claims to be "Putting the *fun* back in funerals" but I would consider this a step rather too far!

Cremation is becoming an increasingly common means of disposal. Many times, I've heard patients declare that their particular fear about cremation is that they "might not really be dead." I am uncertain how comforting Doug's guarantee is when he declares that he will ensure they are dead. Cemeteries are indeed running out of space and more people seem to be adopting the attitude: "when I'm gone, I'm gone." Sadly, many graveyards are magnets for drunken yobs, base enough to deface and vandalize headstones or wreck floral displays and shrines, which have been lovingly tended by families.

I am pleased to say that we have a good working relationship with Doug Graves and his colleagues. He knows though that his calendar will hang in my garage, rather than in the surgery and I know, if he keeps missing his surgery appointments, he'll be counting down his own days.

NEW PREMISES

I attended the opening of a health centre last night. I do not mean that I stood outside at five minutes to eight as the shutters were being raised, but rather I popped along for the ribbon-cutting of a spanking new, city medical practice. Despite knowing the partners at the practice reasonably well, the glossy invitation card curiously came from Pumice Health and Technology (PHaT). I confess to never having heard of this particular organization but this was just one more reason that convinced this inquisitive soul to venture along.

I arrived in good time. Well, at least it was good time when I entered the car park. The new health centre is overshadowed by an even larger bingo hall next door. I had little idea how popular this untaxing evening's entertainment clearly is and circled (the car park not the numbers!) several times, before finally abandoning the vehicle astride a kerb.

The equally brightly lit health centre was no less busy. I had expected a small, informal group but there must have been a couple of hundred people chatting animatedly. I had not been aware it was a black tie affair either and my tweed suit likely gave the impression (and the subtle country aroma!) that I had travelled from beyond the city boundaries.

The great and the good from the medical world were there. I recognized a few professors, consultants and former colleagues and chatted with some of these ageing but familiar faces. We exchanged polite comments about what we had already seen of the pristine building. Long-retired general practitioners expressed bemusement at the apparent need for such space in a way corner shop vendors do at the arrival of huge supermarkets. Smooth-suited but slightly portly fellows from PHaT mingled expertly and effortlessly and were there to answer all questions. All, that is, except those of actual cost. I inquired about the company and the name Pumice. I learned that there are many such companies able to help practices "design and facilitate the construction of purpose built premises." They are available to assist doctors, who are not necessarily business minded folks, to "envisage and realize the future of primary health care." The terminology and jargon tripped of the corporate tongue quite easily. Private Finance Initiative (PFI) I know is rather controversial in our consumer society, where debt and borrowing have no limit but, if properly managed, can enable building projects which otherwise could never have been contemplated. PHaT pride themselves, like pumice stone itself, in being well honed, natural and able to smooth rough edges. Many of their rival firms are named after precious stones but pumice, apparently, implies lesser expense and pretension. I retorted by suggesting I hoped the building material and its occupants were hopefully rather less porous, fragile and dull. In addition, did they know pumice was the product of hot air and effluent?

Before I could be escorted from the building, a chinking spoon on a glass eventually managed to hush the gathered throng. Speeches from proud GPs and senior PHaT representatives followed, detailing how many years the project had taken from conception through to completion, with all the obstacles and mishaps in between. We were then invited to wander throughout the building (I'm sure I was being closely observed) taking in the consulting rooms, reception areas and ancillary staff facilities. Closed circuit TV banks showed the health centre inside and out and I even managed to see a warden carefully place a ticket on my windscreen. A high-calorie buffet awaited us upstairs and a carved ice representation of the building started to melt under the strong lights.

As cynical as I can be and as unimpressed as I was by some of the more exaggerated claims I heard earlier in the evening, I could not help but admire the fabric,design and comfort of these new premises.

I will be returning to our own rather tired, cramped and dimly lit surgery on Monday and wonder if I should suggest we go down a similar route. We would likely lose the character of the place, I suppose, but it seems that is what modern, progressive general practice is all about.

PRACTICE BOUNDARIES

"Please may I stay with the practice, sir," implored Fran Tier. "I've been here all my life and never really bother you." Fran had indeed been registered with us for his two-score years and had been a trouble-free and healthy patient. Looking at his records, he had only consulted us or been brought by his mother on five occasions. The trouble now, was that Fran had moved house. He lost his job as a farm hand at Margins Farm, which lies at the practice periphery. He had secured new accommodation at Beyonder Farm, but this is three miles outwith our designated boundary. In a rural practice such as this, twenty-four furlongs (five-and-a-quarter thousand yards!) may be a relatively short distance but is outwith our range nonetheless.

Practice boundaries are necessary but set, arguably, by fairly arbitrary means. They were often drawn decades or even centuries ago and took into account natural features such as rivers and hills but roads, railways and county divisions were also considered. We have an oak-framed parchment map displayed in the waiting room, clearly demarcating our defined territory. It is far from being a perfect circle, with the practice centrally, but is rather an irregular, amorphous expanse of some three-hundred square miles. This area approximates to that of an average city, as I occasionally remark to my urban-dwelling, diesel-breathing colleagues.

Ours is the only practice in the town and we encompass several villages and hamlets. We do not have any other (satellite) premises. Our area overlaps a little with one or two neighbouring surgeries.

Some patients over the years have expressed disenchantment with us and taken their complaints elsewhere. Conversely, we have inherited others who left (or were asked to leave!) neighbouring practices.

When they move, people can be remiss at informing us of their new details. This may be deliberate or otherwise. It may only come to our attention that a flit has occurred when we receive a hospital letter supplying a different address or when we are asked to phone a patient and her home number has an unfamiliar area code. We are not looking for reasons to get rid of patients or to keep our numbers down, but new patients are always moving into the area and we simply cannot accommodate and accumulate every patient who has ever registered with the practice.

The one group more difficult to be dogmatic about is students. We appreciate that under-graduates go to colleges and universities for only three or four years. We encourage them to register with local or campus based practices but appreciate they may be back home several times each year. There may be ongoing medical or psychiatric problems which benefit from knowledge and familiarity. If a patient is in the middle of complex treatment I tend to agree to him remaining on the list until such time as he can transfer to a more appropriate and local GP surgery. Clearly this could only occur if he was moving a short distance and not to the other end of the country or the earth.

It is also difficult to tell long-registered patients, if they are not moving particularly far, to sling their hook but a line has to be (and has been) drawn. We cannot allow this line to be expanded like an ever increasing circle in a pond.

It would be wrong to imply that practice boundaries cannot be shifted. Factors such as new housing developments or the closure or expansion of establishments have to be taken into account. As a practice, we have to change with the demography and needs of our population, but we cannot allow individuals to determine the area we cover.

Fran felt we were letting him down. He argued that he could

easily hop on a tractor to get to any future appointments. He reminded me that he had never required a housecall, but that wasn't really the issue. People take unexpectedly unwell, such is the nature of an emergency, or become elderly and frail. Exceptions have been made in the past and tragedy or near disaster has been the result.

He was asking if we could roll back the borders and push back the frontiers. Instead it seemed we were pushing back Fran Tier. He did not see it, but it really was for his own good.

NEXT PLEASE

Some three dozen times each day I spring from my chair, stride down the corridor to the waiting room and call breezily for the next patient. (Well, perhaps not quite as enthusiastically as all that!) There is much discussion, debate and breast-beating about appointment lengths in general practice but little investigation of the intervals between these consultations. There is no right or wrong way to scoop the patient from the waiting room and deliver her to the chair facing mine, but I suppose physically lifting is not the ideal means for my back or my patients' dignity. Different practices use different ways of doing this; the geography and lay out of the premises make for such variety. In larger health centres all eyes are glued to scrolling message boards informing which individual from the waiting crowd is next being summoned. Turning waiting rooms into little more than departure lounges I think is rather sterile and impersonal.

Having previously used a bell, buzzer, tannoy and receptionist, we found the most efficient means was to resort to the good old fashioned method of calling the next patient by name from the waiting room door. I say "by name" but one former colleague, concentrating on the condition of his next patient would often absentmindedly announce "Mrs Gallbladder","Mr Pancreas" or something even more awkward to a bewildered audience.

I am not averse to the regular exercise of to-ing and fro-ing. The alternative would be to be stuck in my chair from dawn to dusk. Before penning this article I timed how long it takes me to usher in every patient of the day. I included the time taken to exchange pleasantries and deal with distractions such as bumping into other patients in the corridor or signing prescriptions stuck under my nose by hovering receptionists. It was astonishingly an hour, less the time it takes to boil a kettle. I would not be surprised if Management on the back of this information suggest we use this time more efficiently. They might contend we could start the consultation before entering the room or see more than one patient at a time. Confidentiality would of course forbid this, but some patients do indeed start listing their complaints as soon as they rise from their seat. I suppose, strictly speaking, the consultation does commence in the waiting room. Observation is an important part of medical diagnosis. Mr D'Eaph, attending with wax, may fail to hear my clarion call. Simple repetition may not catch his attention and a nudge from Mrs Q. Wayter seated next to him may be required. Many elderly folks and those attending with bad backs or unsteadiness can take an age to rise, collect their belongings and totter through. This is entirely understandable but there are those who feel the need to assume the "patient role"by launching into coughing fits, holding their sore parts or dragging a leg melodramatically behind, as if to gain validity for their visit.

There are other reasons for delays in starting the consultation proper. Busy people (or those who like to give that impression!) feel the need to continue conversations on their mobile phones. Mums might have legions of children to round up or discover that one is missing or still being sick in the toilet.

Appearing in person at the door numerous times each day does have its other advantages. It is often my best chance to catch the headlines from the newspapers in which people are deeply engrossed. Alternatively, I might notice a patient who attended me previously but has chosen his second or third opinion from a colleague. He would be the one choosing not to make eye contact or shifting uncomfortably in his chair. For me, just one less patient to worry about. At other times, during emergency surgeries when patients are simply allocated the duty doctor, I get to witness the visible deflation when Niamh Erapi discovers it is me she is seeing that day. Others may have checked in but popped out again for a smoke or taken themselves straight to the toilet. Perhaps visible signs of nervousness, but why anyone visiting their doctor is not abashed at smoking immediately beforehand, I'll never know.

The timber door itself is on a heavy hydraulic hinge. Consequently, I suffer a chronic shoulder problem having to hold it open while buggies, wheelchairs, family groups and other exiting and entering patients stream through.

I have always said the entrance to the waiting room is the busiest junction in town. No wonder its carpet needs replaced annually, but I wouldn't have it any other way.

BLOWING ONE'S OWN TRUMPET

When our eminent senior partner, Dr Bodie Aiken, finally decided to hang up the stethoscope we found ourselves needing, for the first time in years, to advertise for a new colleague.

Mrs Mona Lotte, our practice manager, made enquiries about the cost of a few lines in national newspapers and medical journals. We were most taken aback at the expense but accepted the net had to be cast widely in order to capture (I do not like the word "entrap"!) a suitable and competent replacement for the old fellow.

But what should we say and how would we describe ourselves? Might not what we honestly declare be unattractive to potential candidates? Perusing other such advertisements and descriptions was of considerable interest. The given reason for the vacancy in most cases was the opening gambit. Retirement was said to be the commonest reason, followed by emigration interestingly and, thirdly, by moves into other areas of medical practice. Few pieces stated that the erstwhile partner is currently serving time at Her Majesty's pleasure or has run off with the junior receptionist, though what was written in a few cases may have been euphemisms for certain indiscretions. Other terms seemed to be thinly-veiled attempts to cover the actual situation. "Good sense of humour essential" suggested, to us, that conditions were probably so fraught that a certain detachment was necessary for survival. In addition, to describe any medical practice as "busy" might imply that things are so chaotic as to be unmanageable.

Many practices described themselves as: being modern; well-organized; committed; progressive; being situated within a beautiful locale, having an above average income (can 90% of practices really declare this?), forward-looking, friendly, supportive, cohesive and democratic (can patients vote you out, I wondered?)

We did not wish to appear cliched and predictable, suspecting that being economical with the truth would likely see us searching for a replacement in six-months and having to be more circumspect in the process. Besides, we have our own standards.

Once we had settled upon our fairly modest advertisement, we waited for the applications and Curriculum Vitae to roll in. We hadn't promised the earth but had been candid (for the benefit of candidates!) and that was perhaps reflected in the relatively few interested parties. Some applications came from the other end of the country, making no mention of either work or even visits within 200 miles of here. We suspected these were from people who applied in a blanket fashion; everything and everywhere in the expectation something would eventually pop up. We quickly discarded these and studied the resumes of those who appeared to have a more genuine interest.

All applicants seemed to have more than adequate training and suitable experience. We even wondered if some were over-qualified and excessively dynamic, fearing that work in a small market town might not prove sufficiently challenging. It was rather poignant to note that, by comparison, we would not currently stand an earthly chance of securing our own positions. But thank goodness there is more to being the right person for the job than what is documented (and embellished!) on paper. What did amuse us was the part where candidates were invited to describe themselves, their qualities and what in particular they could contribute to our practice and its patients. Terms such as "vastly experienced", "high-achieving", "excellent inter-personal skills" and "supremely motivated and inspirational" were all very well but did not suggest that modesty was one of one's lesser virtues. Three were selected for interview. We felt it fair to have prepared questions and then allow time for more informal discussion. One or two questions were designed to determine how our potential partner might react under the pressure of an average day and a couple of other teasers were set to see if lateral thinking was within their remit.

At the end of the process we were unanimous in who we felt was suited for the job. We know this particular doctor will get on well with our patients and will likely also tolerate us as colleagues!

The other two candidates, we felt, blew their own trumpets just a little too loudly; not quite fitting their own glowing descriptions nor matching what we envisaged.

Dr Horne was just a little more muted and starts next month.

PATIENTS' SURVEYS

As family doctors, we generally enjoy this job of caring that we do and assume it is appreciated by our patients. Previously, we hardly ever gave a second thought to whether our work would stand up to scrutiny or was even of a decent standard. Patients would politely inform us of any perceived shortcomings and we would graciously take suggestions for what they were worth. I think we used to tot up the notifications of complaint against those of thanks and praise. The latter typically outnumbered the former and tended to stick longer in the memory; and the cards remained longer on the shelves.

Recent changes in general practice have not necessarily been for the better and one new stipulation is that we conduct an annual poll of our patients' opinions and comments.

Facing financial penalties if we desisted, a random selection of patients was generated from the computerized practice list and hundreds of letters posted out. In addition, a stack of questionnaires sat at reception for a few weeks and attending patients were invited to complete these as an alternative to reading golf and lifestyle magazines. I may seem a little more cynical than usual but I confess a dislike for anonymized so-called "satisfaction surveys." I have a particular lack of enthusiasm for questionnaires that demand a rating for all "provided services," from "very poor" to "excellent" with the neutral option of "fair."

Never one to readily accept change (especially when it appears to be for change's sake), I see this exercise as a bit of an imposition and really rather misguided. I feel it provides yet another platform for the evolving breed of "serial complainers" who find fault wherever they look, have little comprehension of the workings of day-to day medical practice (or any other organization) and, quite frankly, seem to have rather too much time on their hands. I've observed that people who are satisfied remain quietly contented with the service they receive and those who are not, or simply don't get their own way, are quick to vocalize and criticise without offering constructive advice. My concern remains that "the voice" of the patients may be a rather croaky one, which is biased or simply an unrepresentative one.

Nonetheless, after jumping through yet more hoops and bending over backwards (metaphorically speaking, you'll be relieved to note!) to please our paymasters and the faceless number crunchers, and partly out of curiosity, we sat down to analyse the "data." The findings made interesting, though questionable, reading.

Firstly, the present out-of-hours arrangements was a recurring theme. Recognising that the situation may not be perfect, the expressed desire that "I expect to be able to see my chosen doctor, day or night" is both anachronistic and unrealistic. Even if sleepless on-call rotas once came close to providing such a "personal physician," these days are long gone. Secondly, the length of waits for appointments was also singled out for criticism. This was both the time taken from requesting to obtaining a consultation and the minutes spent in the waiting room, sitting "patiently" (or completing such surveys!) Closer reading of comments showed that some patients refuse to see anyone other than their preferred doctor. No account was taken for periods of leave and little acknowledgement that we always maintain, in cases of genuine urgency or need, patients will be accommodated the same day. Thirdly, our individual consulting styles were called into question. Lack of time, failure to make eye contact, not taking a comprehensive history and not allowing the patient sufficient involvement in decision-making were all kicked-up as points of criticism. Receptionists were described as "like guard dogs" and some other staff members as "unhelpful" and "they don't put me at my ease." And you should have seen the negative comments!

Of course, as difficult as it is to imagine, neither I nor the practice are perfect! We should be receptive to constructive criticism and informed advice and should always strive to improve (but don't expect a woolly mission-statement from me!)

I feel, with the nature of these generic surveys, that replies can be unqualified, factually incorrect or taken out of context. Their design has little appreciation of the life, work and variety in general practice. On the whole, despite the above, we were portrayed quite favourably and achieved most of the rather arbitrary statistical "requirements."

I think most consumers, voters and even patients in today's society are becoming just a little tired and even suspicious of the apparent endless need for target-setting and opinion gathering, all in the name of market research and quality control. The feeling, I believe, is that there is often another agenda-goods to be sold, votes to be won or responses to be skewed and twisted for other purposes.

I'd rather not think of my patients as customers or clients but perhaps I'm just resisting the notion that I'm a simple, measurable commodity (close to its sell-by-date!)

For the moment though, we (and our patients!) seem to be ticking the right boxes.

RACE RELATIONS

One of my mid-morning tasks is to read the day's correspondence. Hospital letters are usually rather dry, informative missives and I scanned such a pile this morning. There was one, however, that stood out. It was from the Surgical department at the infirmary. I had referred a lady on a matter that was beyond my expertise (assuming of course, I have any in the first place!) The typed summary commenced in the usual polite fashion and proceeded to give details of a thorough examination, appending the results of relevant and sophisticated investigations.

The closing paragraph caused me to almost cough my coffee over the page. The doctor wrote that my patient, Mrs Predd (Judith) commented disparagingly about the colour of his skin and enquired whether he might not be better practising in the land of his origin. She had apparently proceeded to denigrate his senior colleague, of similar ethnicity whom, he said, he was relieved was out of earshot. Despite the unsolicited and unwelcome comments, he agreed to review our patient again on clinical grounds, but stated that if she were to vent forth again in such an inappropriate fashion there would be no option other than to "suggest she seeks her future care elsewhere."

I was astonished. Firstly, that this seemingly rational patient should own such opinions and, secondly, after receiving excellent care and attention should feel it necessary to express her beliefs in such an intemperate and inappropriate fashion. I was also annoyed and embarrassed. I wondered whether I should call my hospital colleague to thank him for his tolerance and apologise on her behalf but she really only represented herself, not the practice. If I were to contact him, it would be to say that I had not been aware of her overt racial prejudices. I would be happy to share in any decision as to how best deal with the matter.

This was of course not the first time I have encountered prejudice, racial or otherwise, in my career. My observation is that prejudice rarely comes from those who have contributed much to society themselves. I sometimes listen to patients describe their frustration at finding the doctor in clinic as having been difficult to understand. This may be an actual problem but a melodramatic, lampooning of a thick Pakistani, East European or Oriental accent is unnecessary and really rather foolish. Imitation is not always the sincerest form of flattery.

People seem to forget that Asian, African and other doctors, born or trained abroad, have much to offer the NHS. Indeed, they are often better educated and more competent than their "home grown" counterparts. It may be the glittering prize for graduates from India, Malaysia or Kenya to work in the UK and this is only achieved by passing additional entrance exams, including demonstration of competence in written and spoken English. How disappointing it must be for these doctors to discover a lack of appreciation and even hostility from their patients; the very people to whom they offer their expertise and knowledge.

It should not be forgotten that doctors from abroad were invited to work here during the 1960s when medical staffing was in crisis. The then Health minister, one Enoch Powell interestingly, anticipated a critical shortage of medical personnel and made an urgent appeal for doctors from abroad. Some 18,000 Asian doctors answered his call and soon filling these vacant positions. Many of the GP posts were considered less attractive or less prestigious, mainly ones in inner cities or industrial urban areas. In secondary care, specialist Asian doctors could often only gain access to the more "Cinderella" specialities. One such doctor later said that: "If a job came up the English person would get it first, followed by the Scot, the Welshman, the Irish, the Pakistani, the Indian, the Sri Lankan, the West Indian and the African. This was regardless of qualification-but it meant I knew I would get the fifth job to come up." (And to think I would have taken umbrage at being placed second!) Fortunately, such a pecking order now longer exists, at least not at an institutional level.

I am no more in favour though of so-called positive discrimination where minorities are given preference in order to achieve "balance." This may be well-meaning but again fails to recognise true merit and suitability for a job.

As this generation of Asian doctors approaches retirement, it is predicted that a further import of doctors from abroad may be required. At present a quarter of all UK medical personnel are from the Indian subcontinent and this may rise. If they are of the calibre and have the dedication of their predecessors they should be welcomed with open arms.

Mrs Predd (Judith's) arms, however, will likely be no more open than her mind. After consideration and discussion with colleagues I sent her a letter. I suggested she might wish to clarify why she replaced the more customary words of thanks with hurtful ones.

I expressed my disappointment that she had chosen to embarrass herself, her GP and the hospital doctor.

I doubt my carefully chosen words achieved much and she probably continues to spread her own thoughtless ones. I suspect I'll never know, for she failed to reply, such was the strength of her argument.

MEDICAL STUDENTS

One of the pleasures of general practice is when we have a medical student in residence. Several times each year, a doctor-in-the-making is dispatched from the university to this rural, southerly locale. It usually emerges that he or she asked for a non-urban attachment but was surprised at just how far from supposed civilization they were posted. And so it was recently with Elle Plaitz. Elle is in her fourth year and is normally snugly ensconced with three other medics in her west-end flat. This abode, she said, is within rolling distance of the campus and museums but, more importantly, numerous bars and attractions. A single, "silent as the grave" room in the attic of the cottage hospital was indeed regarded as somewhat of a change.

As a smaller practice, we can only have one undergraduate at a time but look forward to the two months each spends with us. It's fun to hear about their individual stories, backgrounds, interests and expectations of their future medical careers (assuming we don't put them off completely!)

What is poignant for me now is that most of these young people were born after I started working here at the practice. For the whole of their young lives I have been treating and observing (but I hope not taking!) life in this small community.

The young are typically enthusiastic and eager to learn. It is good for students to start by being a "fly on the wall." It allows them to get a flavour of general practice and what survives of traditional family medicine. They often comment at the contrast between how well we seem to know our patients and the general anonymity of those in hospitals. We are keen for students not to be shackled to just one GP during their attachment but rather to spend time coat-tailing and monitoring each of us. We certainly have different consultation styles, according to our personalities and experience. I am sure it quickly becomes clear that I am no academic and practise the art, more than the science, of Medicine.

It can be challenging to be quizzed on decisions we take. Much of what I do is probably at a subconscious level and I would rather try to justify my diagnostic and prescribing habits to a student then to a court of law. It is refreshing to hear a less experienced but literal and unbiased view about what we face daily in surgery and in people's homes. After a week or so of sitting with arms crossed, Elle was invited to change seats with me and see a few patients herself. I became the "fly" and would only intervene if the consultation was drying up or to bring it to a conclusion.

From a patient's point of view, students are often a welcome addition to the practice. About one in ten, however, asked that Elle leave the room as they felt their problem was rather too personal. Confidentiality, of course, is paramount but I think some people would rather not discuss their piles or their domestic crises in front of a stranger, especially one in her early twenties. (Sadly, I was never considered as looking too young during my earlier career!)

Students are set the task of identifying four patients to study in greater depth, as case studies. Most people are only too happy to sit answering questions about themselves for an hour or more. They tend to comment ruefully on how their doctors never seem to have such time and interest any more.

I enjoy motoring around the county on visits and am keen to remind these young city-dwellers what hills and sheep look like. Rather than listening to chat or music on the radio, it is an opportunity to hear what troubles or amuses Elle and her colleagues. I also learn how out of touch I am with music, technology and modern methods of education.

Some time ago, Mrs Moody and I felt we should open our

door to visiting students. I worked away from home during much of my training and greatly appreciated the casserole, conversation and Chianti, when offered. We are happy to share supper once or twice a week and to invite our guest along to local events and celebrations. Some of our former students occasionally drop by and it is always lovely to catch-up and meet their families.

After the student has departed, we are each invited to submit an appraisal to the university. It is a useful way of assessing ourselves as doctors and our desire to pass on what we know to the next generation. Once or twice we have been stung by criticism and had the university wag the proverbial finger at us for a perceived lack of organization or formal teaching. I would much prefer such accusations to suggestions we might have been unfriendly or disinterested. We try to take all comments on board to ensure future students have an even more fruitful and memorable stay.

Last week, after a fine dinner with us at a local inn, Elle said her goodbyes. Once again, we learned a lot and hope, if what she said is true, she did too. She returned to her digs and her next attachment but we hope to hear from her again soon.

JACK FROST

The workload and nature of general practice differs greatly from season to season. If we are blessed with a summer really worth talking about (but we'll blether about the weather anyway!) people feel healthier and are happier about themselves. Come winter however, daylight is short-lived, moods dip and viruses strike. Some wealthier types are able to chase the sun by jetting to their villas in Majorca for a few months, enjoying a perennial summer. For the rest of us, we are subject to our increasingly unpredictable climate and all that it has to throw at us.

I am an ardent supporter of the annual flu jag. It was only a few years ago that there was a strong suspicion it was more a source of ill-health than a prevention. It has pleased me to see, over time, the acceptance of its benefits but some patients still decline it each time around. The argument that "I've never had the 'flu yet, doc, so I'm not likely to get it now" holds no more water (ice?) than suggesting one has never been hit by a bus so needn't bother checking left and right when crossing the road.

The tragedy of winter, here in Scotland and other countries of a similar latitude, is the unnecessary deaths that occur during these months. Older people, in surgery, sometimes express their fears about being "taken by Jack Frost." They might slip on icy pavements and suffer serious head injuries or significant fractures, from which they may never recover. It is estimated that 25,000 elderly people die as a result of cold weather each winter in the UK. It really is sad if people feel they have to make the choice between heating and eating. If they really do have to choose between turning on an electric bar or eating a hot meal there really is a problem, both for them and society as a whole.

But it is not just the elderly who are vulnerable to the effects of freezing temperatures. Young people, perhaps on Christmas nights out and who have overindulged, are underdressed for the conditions and overconfident in their ability to make their own way home, may never make it. Almost every year I read of dog walkers falling into frozen ponds when their beloved pet falls through the ice and rescue attempts prove futile, and fatal.

There is discussion amongst academics of a more wintry disposition about whether Jack Frost originates from Russian folklore or Viking mythology. Reference to him certainly dates back centuries and he is often portrayed as a somewhat villainous and mischievous character. Despite his malevolence and murderous ways, it is he who touches objects including windows, creating the most beautiful ferning patterns. These are as unique as the design of snowflakes and are different each time. Such glass geometry or translucent tapestries are indeed fine to look upon, drawing back the curtains on a bitter January morning, but less attractive on and in a tumbler of water on one's bedside table. False teeth were never supposed to be suspended in blocks of ice!

Winter fuel payments from the government to older people in genuine need are to be welcomed but the most vulnerable members of our communities should be identified. There is an onus on us all to keep an eye on elderly neighbours and family members at this time of year. Whether it is first-footing with a bag of coal or providing groceries during these more difficult times, there is much we can do to keep Jack Frost and his cousin the Grim Reaper away from the door.

DO YOU LIKE WHAT YOU SEE?

I don't know whether, technically, the mirror was invented or discovered but, since someone first caught their reflection in one, the human race has never been the same.

Few houses and bathrooms are without these glassy reflectors. After the waltzers, my favourite fairground attraction is the Hall of Mirrors. It is almost impossible not to be amused when seeing oneself look squashed, twisted or stretched to implausible proportions. As I rarely catch sight of my full-length profile, I usually let others wander by first to ensure there actually is some form of visual trickery occurring. Most of us can laugh at such distortion of our dimensions and falsification of our features but clearly there are those who cannot and, not only that, those who despise the undistorted image staring back at them.

We should rejoice in our diversity and variety but the expectation of perfection and flawlessness has led to a society disgruntled and depressed with itself. I see this in the surgery on a weekly basis. People are unhappy, and are being encouraged to be displeased, with their appearances. Women's, lifestyle and, I hesitate to use the word, beauty magazines show us (well, those who read them!) before and after photos of reconstructive and cosmetic surgery. The resulting "product" is a person supposedly happier and possessing greater confidence. She now "owes it to herself" to stand tall (if she can!), throw her head back, and to go out and demand in life what she truly deserves because, after all, she's worth it!

As the NHS budget gets stretched and squeezed (perhaps using mirrors) to increasing degrees, surgery that is perceived as being more for vanity than necessity is declined. Rightly, children with birth marks or other deformities, though not necessarily life-threatening, are given priority. Women requiring reconstructive surgery after mastectomy are treated rather than those who just feel things are "heading south." The private sector may beckon for those who wish to proceed with their jaw-lifts, tummy-tucks and collagen implants and if they are willing to run the attendant risks, good luck to them, I suppose.

I wonder, though, if it is right for individuals to be made to believe that their nose is rather too large or too hooked; their ears too sticky-outy or their skin too freckly and pale. There may have been bullying at school for appearing just a little bit different and I know the psychological scars from such can be severe. Perhaps advertisers and self-styled fashion gurus are no less than bullies themselves. Even worse, their motive is often financial rather than them being silly kids who just don't know any better.

I am no oil-painting and have been told by Mrs Moody that I stopped spending time on my appearance the day after she replied "I do." I am not suggesting that people should stop trying to feel good about themselves or ought not try to "reverse the ageing process." Almost all women, from a certain age onwards, use hair dyes as well as make-up but chaps are still viewed with a little suspicion, at least around these parts.

What makes me very sad is when a teenage girl attends with her mother with reports of self-harm or other expressions of self-loathing. I gently enquire as to what she would change about herself if she could and am answered with the single word: "everything." Anorexia is both a fascinating and tragic condition. It remains unfathomable to me why these, usually highly intelligent, young people remain utterly convinced they are obese. Furthermore, there is often the stated desire to continue losing weight, regardless of the cost, to themselves and their families.

Of course, the ultimate disappointment in what one might see in the mirror is that of gender identity crisis. There are some people who, from an early age, are convinced they inhabit the wrong body; that they are female and should have been born with only one X-chromosome or male and resent having a Y. I have met patients with such convictions but have yet to refer anyone for reassignment surgery. There are rather lengthy psychological assessments before it is ever agreed to proceed.

I know there is a relation between how one feels and how one looks and how one looks and how one feels, if that statement is not a mirror image of itself. Well-adjusted and contented people may or may not be "good looking" but are at ease with themselves and do not worry about how they, others and the mirror on the wall sees them.

THE LAST PATIENT

I don't suppose we ever know who is going to be our last patient or what problem(s) they will bring. Scribbling on the back of an envelope I calculate that, in my forty years of service (or was it servitude?) to the good people of this community, I have seen some 460,000 patients. That grand total comes about by having seen some patients more than once (and indeed some people several hundreds of times!)

This equates to me having seen all the souls in Edinburgh, and attending to that demanding population would have been rather difficult (or that difficult population, rather demanding!) The majority of this near half-million consultations was of a more formal nature in the surgery but many were conducted in patients' homes. The rest were impromptu consults in the queue at the post office, in the greengrocers or being summoned to relocate shoulders on the sports field.

I certainly remember meeting my first patient at the practice all these years ago. After I discovered that the bell system was considered archaic–I had to summon each person from the waiting room–in came Ian Ischel, my first patient in general practice. Ian did not realize he had this dubious honour (though I suspect the receptionist primed him) but after a few years of training behind me, he was somewhat more than a guinea pig.

To the best of my ability, I have been as professional and competent as I could have been. I think I was as on the ball as I could have been but accept my clinical knowledge was at times no more up to date than my dress sense. As the years went by, my experience broadened; my intuition and gut-instinct grew (well, the gut certainly did!) and my appreciation of human nature and it's relation to illness increased-or at least, I had a greater insight into what I didn't know!

I tried to view each person and every case with clinical detachment and a sense of impartiality and proportion. When practising family medicine, one gets a unique knowledge of a person, his kin and his clan. This is usually helpful but should not detract from the fact that everyone is an individual and should always be seen as such. I remained as discreet as possible and only broke confidentiality when the law or extreme circumstances dictated. I was as decent and mild-mannered a fellow as my character permitted and committed no indiscretions-or at least none to which I would readily admit!

My inefficiency with paperwork was both consistent and predictable. I tended to be distactible and would give each important case my due attention, gladly at the expense of a waiting insurance report. I was sometimes guilty of wishing to be elsewhere or willing to reach the end of a surgery; I won't pretend boredom never afflicted me. Seemingly endless trivial complaints, at times, were close to wearing me down. Occasionally, my confidence was shaken by developments that were quite contrary to what I expected or when I frankly got it wrong. But every week there were several patients who were in genuine physical or emotional need. I'm no better a diagnostician than any other doctor but on the occasions where my intervention or recognition of a problem proved timely, there was no greater feeling or sense of purpose.

I am not a committee man and will not be spending my retirement on boards, though my boundary fence does need repaired. I know democracy and wisdom dictate discussion and debate but I quickly tire of officious people who have no experience or training in the field in which they have influence. Call me old fashioned, if you will, but it should be doctors making decisions that affect patients. Perhaps I should have made efforts to contribute to patients' welfare beyond my own practice.

It may have been said before but remains just as true today; a doctor is only as good as his last patient. He (and increasingly, she) may be the professor of neuro-physiology, may hold lecture theatres spellbound with their erudition and wit and may have patients prepared to wait weeks to be seen (ours often aren't given the choice!) but if she makes a rum decision or accidentally pierces a pulsating artery during surgery the consequences are just as devastating. Practising medicine, with the responsibility it carries, is a great privilege and this should never be forgotten. No-one is ever too talented or too experienced not to make basic errors or oversights and not to learn from them. If one is too arrogant to recognize this, he is not practising medicine with the humility he ought.

Anyway, what's all this talk of retirement? Just because I'm of that certain age when one is expected to lay down the stethoscope and tendon hammer and lift the newspaper and take up lawn bowls. Traditionally, a chap in his twilight years will find himself with ample time to arrange his slides and stamps. But I already tackle the crossword most evenings, throw a jack most weeks and have a system in place for filing my photographs and philately. I feel I've still got something to offer and enjoy what I do and while the powers that be tolerate my continuing presence, I'll continue to warm this chair. For as long as I'm still learning, can help restore the occasional person to better health and still laugh out loud on a daily basis, my patients will just have to be stuck with me a little bit longer.